BURKITT

CANCER • FIBER

By
Ethel R. Nelson, M.D.

Preface by former U.S. Surgeon General, C. Everett Koop, M.D.

TEACH Services, Inc.
Brushton, New York

ISBN 1-57258-093-3
Library of Congress Catalog Card No. 97-61573

Published by

TEACH Services, Inc.
RR 1, Box 182
Brushton, New York 12916

TABLE OF CONTENTS

PREFACE vi

ACKNOWLEDGMENTS viii

APPRECIATION xi

1   MOLDING THE CLAY 1

2   A PROVIDENTIAL DISAPPOINTMENT? 16

3   ARMY AFRICAN ASSIGNMENT 29

4   LOVE FOR OLIVE AND AFRICA 43

5   EARLY YEARS IN KAMPALA 58

6   ENCOUNTER WITH A UNIQUE CANCER 72

7   NAILING DOWN A "LYMPHOMA" 86

8   THE 10,000-MILE SAFARI 97

9   FILLING IN THE GAPS 109

10 THE GREAT VIRUS RACE 120

11 FINDING THE VIRUS CONNECTION 133

12 TAKING A NEW DIRECTION 144

13 TABOO STUDIES 158

14 FORTUITOUS CONTACTS 171

15 MORAL FIBER 181

16 WALKING THE SECOND MILE 191

17 "BURKITTISMS" 210

18 HOW TO HANDLE HONORS 225

19 THE POTTER AT WORK 242

EPILOG 259

SELECTED BIBLIOGRAPHY 261

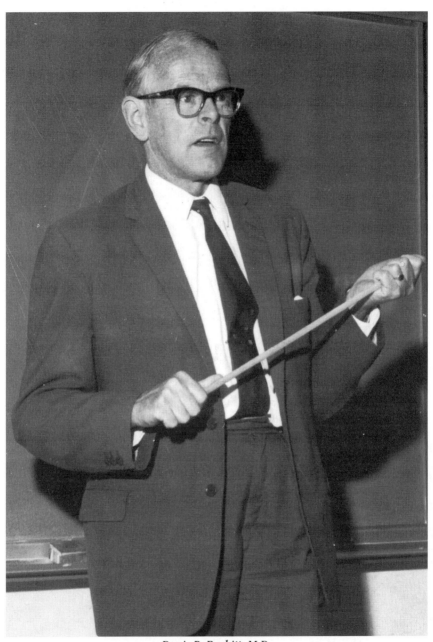

Denis P. Burkitt, M.D.
(Lecturing at Loma Linda University School of Medicine.
Photo from collection of Albert Hirst, M.D.)

DEDICATION

To Olive Rogers Burkitt
More than a helpmeet,
An ever-present inspiration,
The epitome of hospitality,
A Christian counselor,
A best, loyal friend
to Denis

PREFACE

Not many biomedical scientists with training and credentials have had as much impact on health and medicine as Denis Parsons Burkitt. He had no laboratory, no assistants, no high-tech equipment, but just as Benjamin Franklin discovered electricity with a kite, a ball of string, and a key, Denis Burkitt made discoveries that have affected millions and millions of people, especially those who sought control of their diet in line with preventive medicine.

Denis Burkitt's research led to the establishment of a virus-cancer linkage in the childhood disease now known as Burkitt's Lymphoma. He also helped society and the medical community to understand that dietary fiber deficiency is one of the primary causes of many diseases in the industrialized world.

In trying to account for his rather remarkable life, Denis Burkitt was fond of telling listeners that attitudes were more important than abilities, motives more important than methods, character more important than cleverness, perseverance more important than power, and the heart more important than the head.

I would agree that all of these things were instrumental in making Denis Burkitt who he was, but I would also say that Denis Burkitt was at heart and soul a missionary. Whether he was a missionary of the Gospel, a medical missionary bringing his measure of health and comfort to those who were sick and needy, or whether he was preaching the virus-cancer linkage or the story of dietary fiber, he did so with the zeal of a missionary.

I was pleased to be with Denis Burkitt for part of his last major undertaking before he died in England on March 23, 1993. He had come to the United States in

January primarily to receive the Bower Award and Prize for Achievement in Science at the Franklin Institute in Philadelphia. The award consisted of a gold medal and a cash award of $375,000—certainly a far cry from the frugal days of his early research. During his stay in America he delighted his audiences at the Franklin Institute, during the dietary symposium held there in his honor, and at several other lectures he gave, with his usual wit. He wrote me on January 27th and said, "It is far and away the largest sum I have ever handled and since I do not intend to spend any of it directly on myself, it is quite a responsibility exercising a sense of stewardship in the distribution."

That sentence captures the measure of Denis Burkitt and is in keeping with the effort that Ethel R. Nelson has made to bring the reader's attention to this remarkable man and the life he led for others.

C. Everett Koop, M.D., Sc.D.

ACKNOWLEDGMENTS

While a veteran medical missionary in Thailand, I chose expensive medical periodicals with great care. As a pathologist, I particularly treasured the Cancer journal. When I opened the March 1961 issue of Cancer, an article by Dr. Denis Burkitt, picturing African children with grotesque jaw tumors, immediately attracted my attention. The unusual geographic distribution of the tumor described in the article was even more intriguing. Burkitt, I decided, was certainly to be commended for his perceptive observations. I, too, was convinced that the causative agent of this unique cancer must be a virus. When the Epstein-Barr virus was incriminated a few years later, the discovery opened many new phases of cancer study. How exciting to follow the making of medical history, step-by-step!

In 1970, now back in the States, I attended an American Cancer Society meeting in San Diego, where surprisingly the now world-famous Burkitt, with his name attached to "Burkitt's lymphoma," presented a paper on dietary fiber depletion as a contributing factor in colon cancer. How is it, I wondered, that Burkitt has become interested in nutrition? But this was only the beginning, for his name later became nearly synonymous with "fiber."

It must have been about 1974 when the medical staff of the New England Memorial Hospital, where my husband, a surgeon, and I were now practicing, appointed me to help plan area medical programs. Thinking that a daylong symposium featuring advances in nutrition would fill a growing interest, I suggested that, in addition to seeking speakers from the Boston area, we should see if Denis Burkitt would be willing to cross the Atlantic from England for a presentation. Never really dreaming that he would respond in the affirmative, I was highly pleased when he accepted the invitation. I next wrote to inquire if he would prefer to stay in a motel or be housed in our home during his visit. His immediate and certain response was, "In your home, by all means. I always like to save unnecessary expenditure where possible, and I also enjoy the friendliness of a home."

My husband and I met Burkitt at the Boston airport. He no sooner sat in our car than he announced, "I'm Denis, with one 'n'." Before his delightful visit was over, he had introduced us to the Christian Medical Society, where he had also arranged a lecture, and I had interviewed him for an article, later published in a national health journal.

The years rolled by—in fact, about fifteen years. One day I had a phone call from a friend, Dr. Hans Diehl, who asked, "Ethel, wouldn't you like to renew acquaintance with Denis Burkitt? He'll be speaking at my health program in Canada."

"You're tempting me. I'd love to hear him speak again." I added, "He's one person who has lived such an unusual life and has contributed so tremendously to medicine, that surely someone needs to write his biography."

The next day, Hans phoned again. He had startling news, "Ethel, I just phoned Denis in England and told him you'd like to write his biography, and he's agreed. Now you've got to make the trip to Canada!"

Needless to say, I went prepared with a tape recorder and a note pad. When not occupied with his several lectures, at which he appeared to be his old jovial, well-informed self, he related to me his life story. He informed me then that there was a prior biography, *The Fiber Man*, by Brian Kellock. "The only reason I would agree to another biography," Denis explained, "is that I'd like you to emphasize other more important features of my life neglected in this book. I want my family—my wife, daughters, mother and father—given due credit for their inspiration. I want you to feature medical friends who contributed greatly to the success of my endeavors but have remained in obscurity. Most of all, I want to glorify God for His providential leading in my life." My commission had been outlined, and I have endeavored to fulfill Denis's wishes on these three scores, which actually make his life story that much more remarkable.

After returning home, Denis went through his diaries, tape-recording all pertinent events. He sent me his autobiographical notes. His wife, Olive, submitted interesting comments on their courtship, his home and parents in Ireland, her attitudes and observations on the years in Africa, and their family situation and life. Denis wrote his good friends, Dr. and Mrs. Ralph Blocksma, about the project, and they graciously came by for a visit to our home in Tennessee, bringing pictures and relating anecdotes. Letters from Drs. Anthony Epstein, Ted Williams, Jack Darling, and Cliff Nelson added information.

Finally, my sister, Dr. Frances Read, and I made the trip to England, where we spent a week in the rock-solid, historic Burkitt home, enjoying Olive's superb hospitality. I had a rough draft of the manuscript for Denis to peruse for accuracy. Francie spent her time photographing designated pictures tightly glued in multiple albums. (I especially thank her for all the photographic reproductions in this book). One day we called on Drs. Conrad Latto and Ted Williams in Reading, at some distance from the Burkitt village. Another day we devoted to talking with Dr. Michael Hutt and his wife in Wales. These appointments were a highlight, for I could now attach a face and mannerisms to physicians featured in the book.

There were also the memorable visits with the three Burkitt married daughters, who resided with their respective families short distances away. Judy lived just across the street in the tiny village of Bisley. The grounds of her home showed the handiwork of her husband, a talented landscaper. Cassy, as I might have expected, had her father's bubbling personality. She provided precious old letters written by Denis to her in past years and also related humorous incidents. The family picture was completed by a cordial and helpful chat with Rachel.

In January 1993, just a couple of months before Denis passed to his rest, I was privileged to attend, in Philadelphia, the bestowal of the Bower award and medal upon Denis in recognition of his remarkable medical contributions. I was able to meet Dr. C. Everett Koop, who graciously wrote the preface for this biography. I also met Dr. Joseph Burchenal from Sloane-Kettering, who played a large role in the story, and, once more, the Blocksmas.

Working on this biography, corresponding extensively with Denis, and meeting in person his family and many of his co-workers, have been enriching experiences for me. For months I looked forward to receiving his pithy, encouraging notes, usually scrawled in nearly indecipherable handwriting. For me, the unusual Burkitt story is one that should be told, and I have endeavored to do so in the following pages.

I am greatly indebted to Dr. C. Mervyn Maxwell, himself an Englishman, for his careful editing. Dr. Carrol S. Small, a practiced "word-smith," contributed the title and subtitle for the book. Finally, I would like to thank Teddric J. Mohr for his distribution of the manuscript to interested persons, and for negotiating means for publication of the book.

Ethel R. Nelson, M.D.
Dunlap, Tennessee

APPRECIATION

The author wishes to thank Kellogg Company for making the first edition of this book a reality.

Surgeon John Harvey Kellogg, M.D. recognized early in his hospital practice that fiber played a key role in health. His brother, Will K. Kellogg, emphasized health through the production of fiber-rich food products at the world renowned international health spa/hospital, the Battle Creek Sanitarium, and later founded Kellogg Company. The leadership of W.K. Kellogg has resulted in families around the world being able to obtain economical breakfast cereals which are high in fiber. Kellogg Company continues and expands the concern of its founder, that cereals provide a wholesome food high in fiber.

Kellogg Company became aware of Denis Burkitt, M.D., a British surgeon, who for many years was on government service in Uganda, Africa, doing both research and teaching. Dr. Burkitt is best known for his research into the cause of a cancer that was later known as "Burkitt's Lymphoma." During this investigation, Dr. Burkitt noticed the effects of fiber in the diet of Africans versus Europeans. He spent the rest of his life researching, lecturing, and writing on the effects of fiber in the diet and its ability to reverse many disease processes.

Kellogg Company funded the later years of Dr. Burkitt's research in England, providing support personnel, an office, travel, etc. Kellogg's never used its relationship with Dr. Burkitt for anything other than fulfilling its commitment to make consumers worldwide aware of the link between diet and disease, and more specifically, to make the scientific and medical communities, and consumers in general, aware of the important role of grain-based foods (complex carbohydrates) in a healthful diet.

Kellogg Company wishes to pay tribute to a man who required little, yet gave so much, and changed all our lives for the better. Kellogg's hopes that readers will continue to expand their knowledge and understanding of the critical role that diet plays in a healthy lifestyle.

1

MOLDING THE CLAY

Doctor Burkitt caught his breath, trying to hide his shock as he moved closer to the child's cot-like bed. Even though Burkitt was an experienced surgeon, he was unprepared for what he saw as he studied the horribly disfigured face of the five-year-old African boy. Leaning down, he gingerly explored the opened mouth with a tongue blade. "Poor little chap!" he whispered, for massive jaw swellings involving the child's entire mouth caused the teeth to hang loosely from the gums.

Shooting a puzzled glance at Hugh Trowell, the boy's attending physician, who had asked him to consult on the bizarre case, Burkitt looked at the boy again. "Cancer! That's pretty obvious," he mumbled. To himself he thought, *But I've never read of anything like this in medical literature, and I've never seen anything like it in all my eleven years in Uganda, either!*

His sensitive fingers felt for lymph nodes in the child's neck. No enlargements. "Strange," he said to the other doctor, "with such a massive involvement of the jaws, I'd expect the cancer to have spread to these nodes."

Reaching for a large brown envelope on the bedside stand, he drew out an x-ray and held it up to the sunlight streaming through the windows of the crowded children's ward. On the film he saw extensive, expanding tumors of the upper and lower jaw bones that pushed away the teeth, jutting them out at all angles.

"You've shown me an awful mystery today, Hugh. Of course there's no hope for the child." As a surgeon, he wished he could suggest something, operate on something, prescribe something. But he shook his head. With a kind word and a sad pat on the boy's shoulder, he left with the other foreign doctor.

How could Denis P. Burkitt, M.D. know that his whole life had been a preparation for this incident in 1957, or that the rest of his life would be shaped by it? This moment was his *life hinge*. Upon it swung all of his past medical preparation and all of his future—bound up in his inquisitive mind.

Research into this boy's type of cancer was destined to make Burkitt world-famous. The tumor would eventually carry his name as *Burkitt's lymphoma*, and a human-cancer-causing virus—the first ever discovered—would be found in it. Years later, in an entirely different field of medicine, because of his global scientific recognition, the world would listen as he also popularized the role of *dietary fiber* in the common, so-called "Western" diseases.

*****

One of Denis Burkitt's earliest memories was partially obscured by recurring hours when he knew nothing. During World War I, Europeans feared contracting influenza nearly as much as they feared shelling, for the disease's toll was great. Now the deadly influenza virus had invaded the Burkitt home in Ireland. In a darkened room, Denis recalled his mother sitting hour-by-hour at his bedside and his father's inquiry each evening when he returned from work, "Is Laddy better? Any more delirium, Gwen?"

"Oh, Jim, it seems he's either listless or tossing with hallucinations!" His mother spoke in hushed tones, and Denis could hear her rinsing a cloth in cold water. The reapplied compress to his feverish forehead felt so good.

"Water, Mummy, please." He seemed forever thirsty.

"What did the doctor say when he visited this afternoon?" his father asked.

"There's nothing else that can be done, Jim. But we can pray." Denis could hear his parents drop to their knees and plead with God that his life might be spared. Then the fog descended and his parents' voices were far away, and fading.

But one morning when he awoke with his mother sitting by his bed, stroking his forehead, she asked, "Laddy, your fever seems gone! Do you feel better?"

"I'm hungry, Mummy," he said. What blessed words! She bent over and kissed him.

"Laddy, I do believe God must have some special purpose for your life. He's spared you in a marvelous way!" Many times afterwards she used those same words, reminding him that God must have a plan for his life.

Neither of his parents lived to see the fruition of such thoughts. But God did indeed have a purpose for this lad.

*****

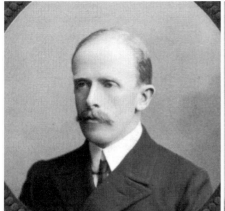

James Parsons Burkitt

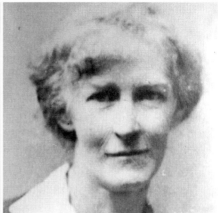

Gwendolyn Hill Burkitt

Only six weeks after Denis's birth on February 28, 1911, James Burkitt; moved the family to their first home estate, fifteen-acre Lawnakilla, about a mile-and-a-half from Enniskillen in northern Ireland. Denis's father, forty-one at the time, was by then an established engineer supervising road construction. When newly graduated, he had taken engineering examinations and become the top applicant for choice positions in three North Ireland counties. He had selected picturesque County Fermanagh with its largest town, Enniskillen, located on an island between two lakes.

As an engineer, he enjoyed a social status above the poor, illiterate cottage dwellers of their village, and so it was expected that Gwen Burkitt have helpers in the home, at least a cook and a maid. A handy man kept the grounds well trimmed and lawns mowed. But having servants didn't mean that either parent was wasteful or idle. Far from it! Once as a lad, Denis observed his mother tearing a bed sheet in two down the middle. Surprised, he asked, "Whatever are you doing, Mummy?"

"The center of this sheet is worn thin," his mother said, having just finished dividing the sheet in half, "but the sides are almost as good as new. Just watch what I do next," She brought the sides of the sheet together and pinned them. "Now, I'll just make a neat seam down the middle, hem up the sides, and we'll have a sheet like new! You mean to tell me that you've never noticed the middle seams in some of our tablecloths? They get the same treatment when they get worn."

But maybe there were some reasonable limits to economy, or so Denis thought in his childish mind. Perhaps this might be the proper moment to bring up a pet grievance. "Mummy, I do wish you wouldn't buy those terrible socks for just five pence (ten cents) a pair," he complained. "They really hurt my feet, they're so rough."

"Laddy, my dear boy, I've never seen blisters on your feet. They can't be that bad!" Gwen Burkitt closed the subject.

3

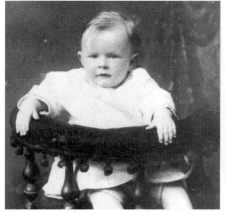 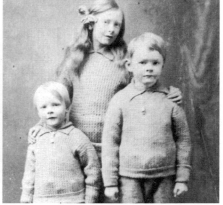

Young Denis Parsons Burkitt   *From left to right: Robin, Peggy & Denis*

His mother wasted nothing, including time. She knit warm sweaters for Denis, his brother Robert, nicknamed "Robin," 18 months younger, as well as for their older sister Peggy. And there were the perpetual darning of socks and mending of clothes as well. But when the household duties allowed her the time, she did exquisite embroidery work, for she loved fine things. As for herself, she liked to look attractive, always changing her attire for the evening.

Denis's father, on the other hand, cared little for his personal appearance. While Gwen Burkitt provided beauty for the home—handsome furnishings acquired as bargains, and lovely flower arrangements—Jim Burkitt saved and securely mended broken household articles, whether the end products were attractive or not.

Christmas rarely brought purchased gifts. Instead, his father spent hours in his workshop fashioning useful toys, little trucks, even bookcases. One Christmas season, Denis found his mother at her writing desk with ink eradicator, busily removing signatures from Christmas cards received the previous year. A perpetual questioner, he asked his usual, "What are you doing, Mummy?"

"These are such pretty cards, I hate to throw them away, so I'm erasing the names on them and putting our names on the cards instead." She looked down fondly at the cards, saying with a smile of satisfaction, "Of course I'm making sure that I send the card to a different friend."

Frugality would become one of Denis Burkitt's lifelong traits, learned early from both parents.

Some of Denis's earliest memories were of his father, before riding off on his bicycle to his surveying work, with binoculars strung from his neck, tramping over the grounds at Lawnakilla, setting bird traps. Jim Burkitt had become one of Britain's first naturalists to band birds, and was thus the first to determine the lifespan of common birds. One of his female robins lived eleven years, a seeming world record at the time.

Denis always admired the resourcefulness of his father who for years carefully plotted maps of the territory claimed by robins and became thereby the ornithologist who first found that every robin has its own specific area. By these observations, James Burkitt initiated the study of territorial behavior of birds. He was active in the British Ornithological Society, for which he wrote several papers,

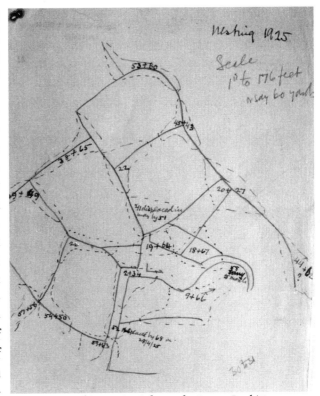

A robin territorial map by James Burkitt

some of them on the identification of bird songs. James Parsons Burkitt would be named, years after his death, as one of seven men who did the most for British ornithology. Interestingly, Denis himself would one day also engage in mapmaking, but his for recording medical observations.

His extended family influenced young Burkitt. When Denis was seven, Uncle Roland Burkitt, on furlough from his surgical practice in Nairobi, Kenya, East Africa, visited the family. One evening, Denis noted fear written on his mother's face when Uncle Roland spun on his chair after peering down his and Robin's throats and demanded, "Can you get a clean sheet, Gwen, to cover the settee?"

"What do you have in mind, Roland?" she asked of her imposing and dogmatic brother-in-law.

"I intend to do tonsillectomies on the boys in the morning," he announced.

Meekly complying with the decision, she quietly said to the youngsters, "Denis and Robin, in the morning, you'll both be taking a long journey, so you'd best get to bed early tonight."

"Tonsillectomies" meant nothing to Denis.

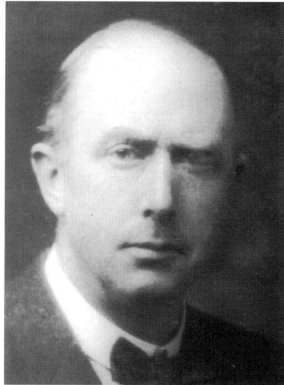

Nairobi's surgeon, Dr. Roland Burkitt

When morning arrived, Uncle Roland brought Denis to the sheet-draped settee in the living room, applied a folded cloth to the boy's face, and dripped chloroform into it. When Denis awoke, he felt cheated, for he hadn't gone on a journey at all. Instead, he was still at home—and suffering from a very sore throat besides.

*****

Rather than send the boys off to school at an early age, Gwen Burkitt arranged for a governess to instruct them at home. Just why his mother was reluctant to send them to the village school, he couldn't understand, but this arrangement suited him fine, for he didn't like books. However, when Denis was eight and younger brother Robin six, they attended a girls' school in Enniskillen. The next year, their mother decided to send both sons to Protora, the prep section of a local public school.

The two boys were close, not only in age but also in companionship, doing everything together. When Denis was given a bicycle by their father, he unselfishly shared it with Robin. So they could ride to the new school together, Jim Burkitt gave Robin a bicycle as well. Every morning shopkeepers in the town knew it must be near eight o'clock as the talkative, punctual, Burkitt brothers pedaled by.

From earliest childhood, Denis cared little for his own appearance or for what people thought of him. There were times when younger brother Robin had to remind him to straighten his tie or brush his hair. Furthermore, school bored him. Only photography, which his father taught him, challenged his creativity.

His parents gave him a Brownie camera when he was ten. With a newly exposed roll of film in hand, he frequently climbed stairs to the dark attic, assembled his trays, and filled them with developer and hypo. After carefully removing the film from his camera in the red glow of a safe light, he passed the strip through the chemicals, rinsed it and hung it up to dry. His excitement mounted as he superimposed the dried film on light-sensitive paper and exposed it to the sun. He watched the black and white prints form while he drew the paper back and forth in the developer. Photography was to become an important lifelong hobby.

One day in 1922, when Denis was eleven, Jim Burkitt surprised the family by arriving at Lawnakilla riding the family's first motorized vehicle, a new Harley-Davidson motorcycle with side car. No more bicycle for his father! Denis watched him build a special seat on the back of the motorcycle for Robin and himself. The shiny new cycle could thus carry the whole family, with his mother and sister riding in the side car, and he and Robin on the improvised rear seat. Denis could just envision their upcoming annual summer trip to the fishing village at Mullaghmore. How grand to roar into the town and see the faces of the amazed fishermen! The trip would now take only hours instead of a whole day. Rather than riding in three separate conveyances—a pony cart, a train, and an Irish jaunting car—they'd simply ride in style across the forty-seven miles of scenic, rolling, green hills to the coast.

That same summer, Denis proved a good enough helper that Jim Burkitt often took him along to help with his highway surveying work. Denis would hold the vertically-numbered staff so that his father could sight it through his transit. Together they would figure the vertical and horizontal angles to insure a level road. At this time Burkitt was constructing his county's first tar macadam (asphalt) highways .

But also during his eleventh year, Denis met with an accident in mid-June.

"Come on, Denis, let's see who can hit the bottle off the fence first." It was a challenge, and several boys picked up rocks to demonstrate their skill. Before long, however, the boys began throwing stones wildly, and then it happened—one hit Denis squarely in the face.

His first reaction was, "You've broken my glasses!" But when his fingers reached up to his right eye and cheek, they came away with blood on them. Dazed, he removed his broken glasses and pulled a folded handkerchief from his pocket to hold over his eye. Unsteadily he picked up his abandoned bicycle, mounted it and headed for home. He was dizzy and frightened. His bicycle wobbled from one side of the road to the other as he pedaled the mile to Lawnakilla. Still holding the handkerchief over his eye, he walked shakily into the room where his mother was sewing.

"Laddy!" she exclaimed, jumping up and letting her sewing fall to the floor. "What's happened?"

"A rock hit my glasses, and my face is bleeding," he said.

"I hope your eye's not injured," Gwen Burkitt exclaimed with trembling voice. "Here, dear, sit down and let me remove the handkerchief and take a look." Gingerly she removed the compress, but quickly reapplied it. "We must go directly to the

7

doctor in town, Laddy. I'll have the pony cart hitched up. You just sit here quietly until I bring it around to the front door."

Within the hour, after examining Denis, the sympathetic family doctor in Enniskillen advised, "I'm sorry, Mrs. Burkitt, but this is a case for the most skilled eye specialist. You must take the lad to Belfast." He then applied a fresh eye patch.

These were frightening words for an eleven-year-old boy! What would be the outcome in Belfast? It was too late to go that day, since the last train had already departed Enniskillen. However, after a restless night, he and Robin, with their father, were on the first train to Belfast in the morning. Before long, they were sitting in Dr. Craig's office. Denis, with some apprehension, looked with his good eye at the various certificates lining the doctor's office wall.

"You've had quite a laceration of your eye, my lad. We're going to keep you for several days here in the nursing home, where I can watch you closely." Turning to Jim Burkitt, the doctor said, "I'd suggest you send a wire to your wife and have her come to be with the boy. I hope we can save the eye. We'll wait and see if an operation is necessary."

With his mother sitting beside his bed the next day, Denis felt better. His father and Robin had returned home. There was little pain, and just lying in bed was getting boring. With his left eye, however, he could see that his mother was worried. Several times she murmured, "God is able, Laddy."

The following day, June 21, when Dr. Craig made his rounds, Denis saw an expression of dismay on his face as he examined the eye. "I'd hoped surgery wouldn't be necessary, Mrs. Burkitt, but it's not healing well. So tomorrow morning, we'll have to operate." He gave Denis a reassuring pat. "It won't be that bad, my boy!"

To help pass the time after the operation, his mother read book after book to him. He noticed his mother was writing a daily account in the diary which she always faithfully kept. Long days passed. Finally on July 5, Dr. Craig called his mother out into the hall to speak privately to her, but Denis could make out what he was saying. "I'm not satisfied with his progress. Mrs. Burkitt. I may need to operate again."

Another ten days dragged by, and on July 15, a second operation was done. For the next several days, he had a recurring fever, and the eye was infected. His mother reassured him again, several times, "God is able, Laddy."

However, after Dr. Craig's visit on July 21, the doctor again motioned his mother to the hall. This time Denis heard him say, "I would suggest you send a wire to your husband to come. We need to talk things over."

The result of the muted conversations between the Burkitts and Dr. Craig was that the eye needed to be removed, as sight in the left eye might be endangered if the infected one were left in any longer. His father had brought him a lovely gift—just right for an eleven-year-old boy—a windup toy boat with propeller. This was some distraction. But, on the morning of July 24, the eye was removed. By evening, Denis was feeling well enough to have several visitors. Jim Burkitt brought his son another wonderful present, a steam engine.

"How much did it cost, Daddy?" the boy asked, amazed.

"It was expensive," his father admitted. "It cost 25 shillings ($6.25). Here, I'll show you how it works. If we put water in it and burn some methyl alcohol in here, the little engine will produce steam which will activate the engine, and turn this wheel."

During his hospitalization, Denis frequently noticed tears in his mother's eyes. However, for him the ordeal was not that bad. In fact, there were additional compensations.

For a boy of eleven, his most vivid memories of the whole affair were the unique gifts showered upon him. Another gift from his parents was a Meccano construction set, which he learned cost eleven shillings ($2.75) and came with a windup motor to mechanize the structures he built. Never had Denis's parents spent this much money on presents! He was so impressed with their extravagance, he would never forget the exact cost of each gift.

Best of all, Denis's wealthy uncle, Sir Alfred Sherlock, who was married to his mother's younger sister, presented him with a 1A Kodak folding camera. Denis estimated it must have cost at least £ 2 ($10.00). It was a big improvement over his Brownie, with distance and speed to set. This camera would serve him well for the next thirteen years.

Finally, on July 31, after a full six-weeks hospitalization, he was allowed to return home. How great it was to be back at Lawnakilla with Robin and Peggy again!

When fall and school time returned, Gwen Burkitt enrolled both sons in a reputedly good school for boys in Holyhead, North Wales. It would mean their separation from the family for most of the year. Denis found that only 22 boys attended the school, where the chief goal of the head master seemed to be to toughen up the youngsters. One requirement, which Denis questioned, was that the boys were to wear white shorts year-round, regardless of the weather. The youngsters also had to take a cold bath each morning. They soon learned to swish in and out of it.

Denis was not an outstanding student, doing well only in mathematics. However, he won a prize for his photography, learned a bit of carpentry, and made a wooden tray which he would use for decades. At the close of each term—Christmas, Easter and summer—both boys looked forward to their unaccompanied trip back home across the Irish channel. Arising early in the morning on shipboard, they raced to the deck to see the welcome green hills of their Emerald Isle.

Denis alone next entered the Dean Close School "with a Christian emphasis" in Cheltenham, England. He still didn't particularly enjoy his classes, for he excelled in nothing. He was shy, and it was rather a lonely time. He could hardly wait until Robin joined him the following year. The brothers never competed with each other, in fact Denis was at the finish line to congratulate him when Robin won his first cross-country run. When Robin won several other races, Denis would rejoice with him, saying, "Another cup to add to your collection!"

"I like to run, but you're great with the signal flags, Denis," Robin said generously.

"You're the one to get the good grades, too, Robin. I don't find the studies as interesting as you do," Denis apologized.

Thus the years passed. Each Sunday, the school's one hundred twenty students duly wore for church services their required Eaton jackets, flat, straw hats and striped trousers, the first long trousers Denis and Robin wore.

*****

In 1925, when Denis was fourteen, an event of greatest importance took place. The family moved to a property, "Laragh," five miles from Enniskillen. Larger than Lawnakilla, Laragh had approximately twenty-five acres and a five-bedroom house with a sitting room, dining room, study and kitchen.

As an engineer, Jim Burkitt was especially interested in the Petter pump which supplied water for the bathroom and filled a large tank with about a week's ration. "Our water supply will last if we flush the toilet sparingly," he advised. "Another thing: don't use too much bath water in the tub. It shouldn't cover the legs." Bathing was a weekly affair, and in the summer, swimming in the lake kept the boys clean.

"A diesel engine will periodically charge large batteries to provide power for electric lights!" he informed them, and paused to hear gasps of approval from the family. "In spite of this convenience, however, we must still use oil lamps, especially if we're in a room for any lengthy session. One other thing: we must remember to switch off the electric light the moment we leave a room." The family grasped these instructions well, for austerity had always been ingrained and expected of each member.

One reason for Jim Burkitt's thriftiness was that his father, Thomas Henry Burkitt, although having a young family of seven children, had voluntarily abandoned the Anglican Church to become a Presbyterian minister. The change proved a great sacrifice, not only in prestige, but also in financial security. As an itinerant Presbyterian minister with a revolver in his coat pocket, Thomas Burkitt rode his horse around Catholic West Ireland, working for a pittance. But with their father's example of penury and dedication, several of his children had, through frugality and perseverance, become professionals in various fields.

There was Denis's mysterious oldest uncle, Robert Burkitt, who left home at fifteen and never wrote other than to send money. After graduating from Harvard University in the United States, Uncle Robert Burkitt, a young adventurer, joined a museum expedition to Guatemala. He remained all his life in Central America. The saying there was, "Burkitt came to tea and stayed thirty years." Becoming an archaeologist and an expert on the Mayan culture, the artifacts Uncle Robert discovered were later displayed in a Philadelphia museum. Uncle Roland was in Africa, and two other paternal uncles likewise spent their lives in a foreign land, both becoming distinguished in the British Colonial Service in India.

The Burkitt's move to Laragh meant a change in church affiliation, with the family now attending a country church at Trory; a short way down the road from their new home. As part of the "gentry," they occupied church pews in front of the laboring class. An alcove at one side accommodated the "lord of the manor" whose family, Denis observed, didn't sit with the rest of the congregation. This high-ranking gentleman had the privilege of reading the lessons aloud each Sunday.

Denis and Robin loved the location of Laragh, for they kept a small rowboat on a river only a half-mile from home. Frequently, in the summer, they hiked to the river with their oars and a haversack containing lunch. Rowing down the river to Lough Erne, they made stops on several small islands in the lake. Homemade bread, a can of sardines, and fruit from the orchard added to the pleasure of these daylong adventures. Summer also invited bicycle excursions—once a fifty-mile trip to the west coast of Ireland with the boys sleeping overnight in a small makeshift tent. Best of all, these simple outings cost very little.

*****

When he was sixteen, Denis was confirmed in the Anglican church with the rest of his class at the school. "Now don't grease your hair," the head master warned them that Sunday morning, "or it'll get on the bishop's hand when he places it on your heads." Church attendance was a requirement which Denis always observed without much thought and with no real commitment. It wasn't until his first year at the university that he would begin to think seriously about spiritual matters.

Through the years, the brothers discussed at length what courses they should take at the university. Of two things they were certain. First, Denis insisted, "We're not quite sure what we will do, but whatever we do, we will never be doctors or dentists! We'll wipe that idea out completely."

The other certain decision was that they would matriculate at Trinity College, Dublin. Denis had been helping his father lay out roads for years and mathematics was his best subject, so it was only natural for him to zero in on engineering when it came time to enroll at Trinity. He found that since few young men in 1929 could afford the fees to go to college, there was little competition for acceptance into the university where he began the engineering course. But even in his own opinion, he thought of himself as rather an unpromising freshman.

During this first year, Denis roomed with a medical student with whom he had little in common. They shared with two other students a sitting room heated by a coal-burning open fireplace. To save money, they cooked their stereotyped bacon-and-egg breakfasts on a gas ring. The atmosphere was anything but homelike, with their toilet across the court. Baths, in a separate building, opened only on Saturday. Fortunately a cold water tap just outside their door supplied their jug with water, while a tin basin served for interval washing.

At the university, Denis found his studies tolerable; however, he was still not motivated enough nor did he study sufficiently hard to make a reasonable standing in his engineering class. But some remarkable changes in attitude took place during his second term. A fellow student approached him one day with an invitation.

"Why don't you come to our Number Forty meetings?" he asked.

"Number Forty? What's that?" Denis asked.

"Sorry, I thought you might have heard of this Christian organization," the student apologized. "We have informal Christian meetings every week. The organization's odd name originated from its first meeting site in Room Number Forty of the college residences. So the meetings have always just been called 'Number Forty.' "

"Tell me more," Denis asked, somewhat uneasy.

"Well, shortly after World War I, several older students who'd been in the war gathered in this room for Bible study and prayer," Denis's friend explained. "Because these older students had experienced war terrors in the trenches, they'd learned to trust God completely and were dedicated Christians. The fellowship they founded grew in numbers through the years and has been a source of inspiration to young men here at Trinity. Many students have made lifelong commitments to mission service."

With this introduction to "Number Forty," Denis began attending and found in the meetings a new and unusual fervor as students shared their Christian faith. After attending several gatherings, he was challenged by an older student. "What do you believe is Christ's claim on your life, Denis? Have you ever responded to Christ's sacrifice for you?"

Denis was momentarily stunned. Profoundly embarrassed, his face burned with shame. Finally, with the young man's eyes fixed intently on him, he stammered, "To be honest, I really don't know. I'm ashamed to say I haven't given it much thought."

How could he give a spontaneous answer to such a bold question? As he considered the disturbing query, Denis knew he had little understanding of the Christian life. What did "being a Christian" actually mean?

He realized if someone had asked him to describe, at this point, the attributes of a Christian, he would have responded, *Oh, I suppose regular church attendance, participation in holy communion, and a fairly acceptable behavior. That should give one at least a 60:40 chance of someday being admitted to heaven.* As he thought about it, he sensed his whole religious philosophy was shallow, works-oriented and without any real understanding of Christ's earthly mission.

After this encounter, Denis became more conscious of God. He determined to study the Bible as a learning adventure rather than as a tedious task. How grateful he became that this young man had had the courage to face him with a personal challenge. For the first time he learned about having a "Quiet Time" with God—a time for personal worship, thought and contemplation of what the Bible's message was for him. Observance of this daily devotional time would henceforth become his lifelong practice for gaining spiritual strength.

In "Number Forty" Denis made new friends. These were serious young men who had the assurance of acceptance with God based on what Christ had done in their behalf. Never had he met this type of faith, and he eagerly sought it for himself. Soon he felt a sense of purpose and direction to his life. He wondered how he could have drifted so aimlessly before.

Does God have a plan for my life? he pondered. His prayers changed as he earnestly searched for God's will, especially about his college course, which had proved so unstimulating. *Does the Lord really want me in the engineering course? How could I serve the Lord as an engineer? Is this the life work I'd really enjoy?* Many questions pressed upon his mind as he tried to determine what God would have him do. *Could it be providential I'm sharing a room with a medical student?* Denis began examining his roommate's medical volumes. He had to admit they did look more interesting than his engineering books.

Now he prayed much about the possibility of becoming a doctor. How would he know God's intention for him? He had doubts about his suitability for medicine, especially since the one class he was almost failing in his engineering course was chemistry. However, in spite of this, he determined to take the entrance examination for the university's next class of medicine. Not only did he spend more time on his knees praying for divine help, but he also earnestly studied for the test.

A few days after he took the examination, Denis held in his hand the envelope with the testing results. With trembling fingers he ripped it open. There it was! Scarcely able to believe what he read, he found he had not only passed the medical entrance examinations, but excelled. He was even near the top of the applicants on the chemistry section!

Maybe God is smiling on me, Denis rejoiced. *This must surely mean God wants me to study medicine!*

He already had certain attributes and character traits, learned in childhood or possibly even transmitted in his genes, that would contribute to the success of his future endeavors. He was keenly observant and had a natural curiosity. His modest self-reliance and insight, accompanied by inborn humility, good humor and frugality, would carry him far. But above all, he was newly nurturing a deep trust in God and His providential leading.

Amazingly, with this decision to study medicine, his personality blossomed. Heretofore a rather shy fellow, he gradually became an outgoing, friendly, confident person. With his new commitment to Christ, his life had taken on purpose.

But what would his parents say? His father was obviously proud that he was following in his steps, taking the engineering course. And in the eyes of his thrifty parents, the money already spent on tuition must have seemed formidable. How would they look upon his starting over in a new discipline at Trinity?

After his first year of college, Denis returned home to Laragh, wondering how to break the news to his parents. When his father invited him along to inspect a new road under construction, Denis felt he had an ideal opportunity for a quiet talk about the subject. However, as mile after mile disappeared beneath the tires of his father's 1928 open-touring Citroen, he still was unable to broach the matter.

Now, as night drew on, they turned into the home grounds of Laragh. Cheery house lights spilling out over well-kept lawns did little to settle his anxiety. Even the tempting aroma of the evening meal, just placed on the dining-room table, failed to ease his mind.

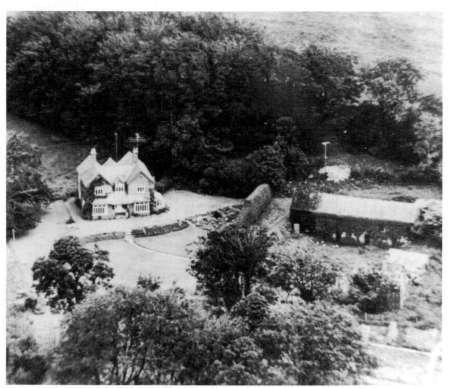

Laragh, with surrounding grounds.

After supper, Denis knew he could delay no longer. With a vague hope that his parents would understand, he hesitated and then, taking a deep breath, blurted, "Daddy and Mummy, I hope you'll understand, but I'd like to change my university course from engineering to medicine!"

Only the cook's vigorous pan-scraping in the adjacent kitchen broke the sudden silence in the room. Denis glanced at his mother. Her eyes registered shock. Scarcely daring to look at his father, he detected disappointment imprinted on the drooping corners of his mouth. He also noted, with increasing discomfort, the rising color in Jim Burkitt's face.

2

A PROVIDENTIAL DISAPPOINTMENT?

No one spoke for what seemed to Denis a full minute. He looked down at his empty plate, waiting for the verdict. When he glanced up, it was just in time to see his mother's astonishment vanish and an exuberant smile light her face.

"I suppose, then," she said, "that someday my son will be called Doctor Denis Burkitt!"

Their eyes met and there was immediate understanding. Hope flickered in his heart. But Denis realized that his father was the final authority in the family and waited rigidly across the table for his answer. As he pushed back a lock of sandy hair, he felt moisture gathering on his forehead. Knowing his father well, he tried to read his thoughts. *Is he disappointed at my not wanting to follow in his footsteps as an engineer?—or is he considering the wasted expense of my first year at Trinity College?*

Jim Burkitt looked at his son, now taller than him by half-a-head, and cleared his throat. "Laddy," he began, being a man of select words, "it's your decision and your life." He even managed a gentle, knowing smile.

Just hearing the old endearing name, so seldom used now, brought a sudden rush of relief. He should have known his parents would agree, but as their elder son, he hadn't wanted to disappoint them in any way. Did he see in the fond gaze of Gwen Burkitt's blue eyes a confidence not previously expressed? She reached over and gave his hand a squeeze, repeating, "Doctor Denis Parsons Burkitt!"

Denis looked across the dining room to a metal case which enclosed from view a fore-and-aft ceremonial hat with a plume of black feathers. He knew the inscription

16

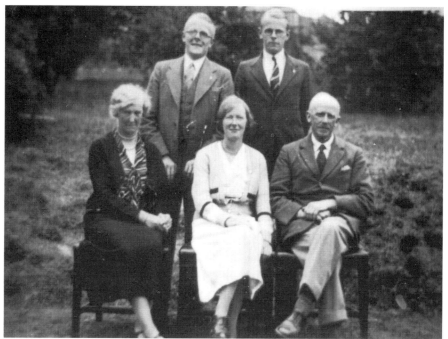

The Burkitt family from left to right:
Gwen Burkitt, Robin, Peggy, Denis and Jim Burkitt.
Circa. 1933.

on its brass plate read: "Dr. W. R. Burkitt, 48th Regiment." Tossing his head in the direction of the memento, he remarked, "*There* was another Doctor Burkitt."

With a touch of pride, Jim Burkitt folded his linen napkin while reiterating the familiar information about the hat. "Yes, that hat belonged to one of your forebears, Denis, a surgeon in the Crimean War."

"You won't be the only doctor in our family, you know," added his mother. "There's my brother, Ernest, as well as your Uncle Roland in Africa."

"Oh—Uncle Roland!" Denis grinned broadly, thinking of his father's brother. "I'll never forget his visit when I was seven."

"Nor I!" she smiled at the remembrance. "I was so frightened when he examined your throat and then Robin's, demanding that I get a clean sheet to cover the settee. I couldn't imagine what he had in mind."

"Uncle Roland's later visit here at Laragh really left me puzzled though," Denis recalled. "Remember when he asked Robin and me, 'Tell me, boys, how many meanings of the word "and" are there in the book of Leviticus?' "

His father laughed. "That's just like Roland. I don't think he meant it as a joke, because he's always had a fascination with words. He never did tell you the meanings of 'and' in Leviticus, either, did he?" It would be more than twenty years before Denis would learn the answer to his uncle's riddle.

Their after-dinner conversation having ended, the family pushed back their red-leather-upholstered chairs and left the dining room to enjoy more comfortable seating in the drawing room.

On this early summer evening at home after the long months at Trinity, Laragh seemed extra special to Denis. While his mother picked up her embroidery and his father a magazine, Denis walked around the drawing room, looking at old familiar objects. With more maturity and purpose than before, he examined these items as though seeing them for the first time. His gaze rested on a small etched portrait of a stern-appearing gentleman with a large wig and a white clerical collar. Stepping across the room to examine it more closely, he next drew out a smooth, leather-bound volume titled, *Burkitt on the New Testament* from the black, lacquered bookcase beneath the picture. After carefully turning a few yellowed pages, he closed the book and looked again at its author framed above the bookcase.

Replacing the book, Denis pulled another volume from the shelf, blew the dust from the top edge and examined the title page: *Sermons of James Parsons of York*. It was dated 1830. Putting the book back on the shelf, he picked up a polished mahogany box and read the inscription on its shiny silver plate:

> This box containing a Purse of one hundred Sovereigns (about
> $500.00) was presented to the Rev. James Parsons by a number
> of his Friends on the completion of the twenty-first year of his
> Ministry in the City of York; as a mark of their high estimation of
> his personal and ministerial character. July 19th, 1843.

His parishioners must have loved Daddy's maternal grandfather, decided Denis. Both Daddy and I got our middle names from him. It's interesting that there are not only doctors, but several ministers as well among my ancestors. Never before had the fact that there were both clerics and physicians in his ancestry seemed significant to him.

*****

As succeeding months and years followed, medical school for Denis was pure joy, and five years passed rapidly. In a class with about a hundred male students, three people stood out: the two girls and an African, Cofie George from Ghana. Denis and Cofie George became instant friends, and it was not long before he invited the African to a holiday at home with him in Enniskillen.

Never before had the residents of this North Ireland town seen a black man, and to Denis's enjoyment, Cofie George made a sensation when introduced to children in the surrounding schools where Denis took him. Pulling down one of their world maps, the African would show the wide-eyed boys and girls his country of origin.

In Denis's second year of medicine, brother Robin repented of his earlier rash decision never to become a doctor and joined Denis at Trinity. Their lives again closely intertwined as they not only studied but roomed together.

During his medical school days, Denis remained active in the "Number Forty" Christian Union. Once, at an evening gathering, a medical student, Jack Darling, visiting from the Belfast Christian Union, gave a talk. After the meeting, Denis felt a tap on his shoulder.

When he turned, he was face-to-face with Jack Darling. "You're Denis Burkitt?"

"That's right," Denis replied.

"Some years ago, my dad and I met your father in Enniskillen," Jack explained. "Since the name of 'James Burkitt' is widely known in ornithology circles and my dad's also a keen bird man, he was anxious to meet your father, who was kind enough to take us to bird haunts around Enniskillen. He also took us to the islands of Lough Erne, where I remember there were thousands of seabirds nesting."

"How was it I never met you then?" Denis asked.

"You were away at school in England at the time; so finally now, after all these years, I get to meet you," Jack finished. He had no idea that many years later, they would work together closely. Jack Darling was but one of several enduring friendships Denis made through the "Number Forty" fellowship.

As graduation time drew on, Denis could never have guessed, a mere six years earlier, that he would finish second in the 1935 Trinity Medical School class, earning a Bachelor of Medicine degree. As a result of his high class standing, he hoped for a resident appointment at Adelaide, his teaching hospital. However, this desirable appointment was handed to a student who had served the college well by his athletic prowess. As it turned out, Denis's first six-month assignment, a "house job in surgery" at the Chester Royal Infirmary, led to new close and lasting friendships. Guy Timmis, a resident surgeon from Liverpool, was destined to become another lifelong friend.

Filled with missionary zeal during his first clinical assignment, Denis began handing out Christian tracts in the Chester hospital wards. His efforts, however, did not go unnoticed. Before many days had passed, his chief surgeon spoke to him privately. "Your activity, Dr. Burkitt," the doctor warned, "is quite inappropriate. Any further distribution of the material will result in your immediate dismissal." This reprimand, forever remembered, was an embarrassment to Denis, who had hoped to fit some profitable Christian endeavor into his medical routine.

For the first time, as a resident physician at Chester, Denis was earning a meager salary. With his own money jangling in his pocket, he decided that the Kodak given him by an uncle following the loss of his eye when he was a lad of eleven had served him well, but that he really should have a new camera. After carefully saving every shilling for a while, he entered a shop and examined one camera after another until he was satisfied that a Zeiss was just what he needed. It was a wise selection, and it would serve him successfully for many years to come.

At this time, postgraduate surgery training in various English hospitals was for six-month appointments. After spending the following six-month period in the Adelaide Hospital in Dublin, he found the summer of 1936 free of assignment. A friend approached him with an idea which appealed to both his love of adventure and his missionary aspirations.

"Why not go with me on a short jaunt to Spain, where we can work with the Spanish Gospel Mission?"

"What would this involve?" Denis asked.

"First of all, we'd have to pay our own way to Spain, and once there, we can get Christian tracts to hand out."

How better could he spend his interlude between assignments? Denis agreed. Since the two young men were on strict budgets, they shipped out from Belfast to Liverpool by the cheapest means—steerage, an accommodation usually reserved for cattle drivers. Laden with tent and belongings, Denis and his friend next boarded a small cargo ship plying between Liverpool and Bordeaux on which they were the only non-crew persons aboard.

Upon arrival in the northern part of Spain, they found an unusual place to camp, under the grandstand at a football field. They had been in Spain only a week, however, when the Spanish Revolution erupted and the British consulate warned them to get aboard a British destroyer with other evacuating refugees. Having been able to pass out only a few tracts, they left on this destroyer for a free passage to Bordeaux. Disappointed at having their plans thwarted, they caught the same little cargo ship headed back to England on its return circuit. They had made the round trip in only two weeks, but with an outlay of fourteen, hard-earned pounds ($70.00)!

Since his next appointment in the fall was still two months away, Denis accepted a temporary job in Wales working for a doctor who wanted a substitute while he vacationed. The £ 8 ($40.00) a-week arrangement was Denis's first experience in the private practice of medicine. He quickly learned its secrets, when the older physician took him into his "pharmacy" and carefully explained, "I have here aspirin in three colors—white, green and pink. I use different colored tablets depending upon the ailment. It's important that you don't mix up the colors for the patients." The doctor opened the record which he was holding in his hand. "You see, I've clearly noted the color prescribed in the patient's record."

This seeming bit of dishonesty on the part of the physician was possibly excusable, Denis decided, since there was little medicine of real efficacy, other than morphine and digitalis. Adding to his lack of confidence in being a relatively new medical graduate, he self-consciously imagined that the villagers must be considering him a mere youngster as they left with their little packages of white, pink or green pills.

His autumn appointment in ear, nose and throat surgery at the Preston Royal Infirmary was disappointing, for he really hated the kinds of operations performed. Perhaps his dislike had begun when his Uncle Roland had done that tonsillectomy so many years before!

By contrast, his year spent as a resident surgical officer in the Poole Hospital, Dorset County, was a happy challenge, for he was responsible for all the surgery, including orthopedics. The other resident, a Scot, Conrad Latto, was fortunately in charge of all the ear, nose and throat surgery, as well as gynecology and internal medicine. Many years later, they would renew their friendship and travel together in India and Africa looking for disease patterns in populations.

He was pleased to find that evening prayers for the patients were an accepted routine in Poole, so he volunteered to take these meetings. Many times patients expressed how much they appreciated his short services. Denis's agreeable assignment in Poole made him think seriously of specializing in surgery, as well as consider a future medical missionary appointment.

The year 1937 marked another milestone. Denis really needed better transportation than a bicycle or a public bus, so he bought his first automobile, an eleven-year-old Austin-Seven touring car, for the remarkable price of £11 ($55.00), even less than the cost of his Spanish trip. Since the car had no self-starter, Denis had to insert a crank under the front grill and give the handle several quick, hard turns to start the engine. He could now easily visit and have a meal with his paternal Aunt May who lived nearby. Her home was to become a welcome haven in months and years to come.

After spending two years in surgical training, Denis felt ready to try the examinations for the Royal College of Surgeons of Edinburgh. His friend Guy Timmis joined him in Edinburgh for three months of intensive study before taking the tests. With this fellowship goal in mind, Denis had put money aside for the fees. He calculated that £100 ($500.00) would be a legitimate expenditure, to

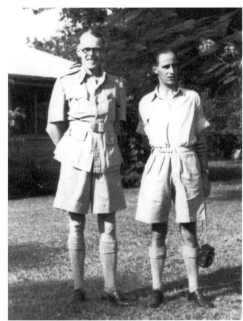

Denis with Guy Timmis. Circa. 1947.

21

include not only the examination fees, but study tuition and living expenses. By sharing room and board with Guy, he figured the budgeted funds should be enough.

So the first business was to find suitable, inexpensive housing in Edinburgh, since both were on strict budgets. After a week in one boarding house, Denis began to calculate, "Really, Guy, our lodgings here are a bit too expensive. Even though three meals a day are included, I think two pounds, two shillings ($10.50) a week is too much. Our finances won't stretch far enough."

"We can do better, I'm convinced," Guy agreed. "I heard of a 'Meadow Place' where we can get the same accommodations for one pound, five shillings ($6.25) a week. Let's make the move."

Each evening they studied together in their new lodgings after spending the whole day in surgical instruction with a tutor. Sundays, however, they took off, attending the Church of Scotland during their stay. Sunday afternoons, the two aspiring surgeons spent taking long walks in the flowering hills around Edinburgh.

Finally the testing time came. The written and oral examinations lasted several days. When the grueling experience ended, Denis thought they deserved a few days of relaxation at his Aunt May's home in Poole. It was while there that a telegram from Denis's parents arrived. He opened it with a prayer, knowing that they were forwarding the results of the exams, and read:

CONGRATULATIONS. DENIS THROUGH. GUY FAILS.

It was with difficulty that Denis broke the news to his friend who, with him, had worked and studied so hard. Guy realized, however, that he'd had trouble in the oral examinations and was not surprised at the results. Denis, having had more surgical experience than Guy, had had an added advantage. Although disappointed, Guy did not for a moment begrudge his friend's success.

Now with his fellowship in the Royal College of Surgeons (F.R.C.S.) in hand, Denis had to decide what he should do next. Should he continue with further surgical training? *I need time to think and pray*, he decided. *I need time for reflection to learn what God intends for me to do*. So, desiring a voyage where there would be few duties, Denis took a job as a ship's surgeon on a cargo vessel to Manchuria. He figured that on board ship he would have time to sort out his future, see something of the world, and make a bit of money—£ 12 ($60.00) per month.

His only assignment was caring for the crew's medical emergencies. While at sea, one of the ship's officers came to Denis with a violent toothache. Knowing little about dentistry, he examined the man's mouth but saw no obvious cavity. After tapping on each tooth, he decided which one to extract to alleviate the pain, and administered Pentothal as an anesthetic. With the man relaxed and unconscious, Denis pulled the tooth, only to find a deeply hidden cavity in an adjacent tooth, no doubt the real cause of the pain. Too late, having extracted the wrong tooth, he realized the diseased one must also come out.

His voyage continued past Palestine, Port Sa'id, across the Indian Ocean to Port Swettenham in Malaysia, then to Singapore, Hong Kong and Shanghai. At each port, Denis looked up Christian churches or local missionaries. On Christmas day, he asked the captain if he could conduct a special service aboard. But the captain was not a Christian, and wouldn't permit it. This refusal reminded Denis of his chief surgeon at the Chester hospital, who forbade the distribution of religious tracts.

Other than finding Shanghai's harbor crowded with Japanese battleships, Manchuria so cold that water in his shaving mug froze overnight, and a major engine breakdown with repair in a rough sea, the voyage was relatively uneventful. This trip was exactly what he needed to sort out his life and consider future plans.

By the time he left the ship, March 3, 1939, Denis had decided on a course of action. From his Quiet Time reading of Proverbs 3:5,6 and Psalm 32:8–10, he knew that the Lord had a plan for him: "Trust in the Lord with all your heart, and lean not on your own understanding. In all your ways acknowledge Him, **and He shall direct your paths.... I will instruct you and teach you in the way you should go**; I will guide you with My eye." He had settled on going overseas on a self-supporting basis, rather than under some missionary society. To accomplish this goal, he decided that working for the British Colonial Medical Service could be a means not only of support but of a desirable overseas location as well. To his way of thinking, he had also solved the problem of where to serve. He remembered his old friend Cofie George, now living back in Ghana. He would plan on going to West Africa.

That very day he called at the Colonial Office to procure books and pamphlets detailing the office's overseas medical assignments. He poured over these to learn what he could about this branch of foreign government service. After all, had not his Uncle Roland practiced medicine in East Africa, and two other paternal uncles served with distinction for the British Colonial System in India? Foreign professional service was not new to the Burkitts.

In the meantime, he felt it wise to continue his surgical training, even though he now held credentials as a surgeon with his fellowship in the Royal College of Surgeons. So he applied with confidence for a house surgeon position at the Winchester hospital. Strangely, the hospital turned down his application. His immediate reaction was, *Why is God leading me in this way?*

The Prince of Wales Hospital in Plymouth, however, accepted him without question for a six-month period. He would be the resident surgical officer, the senior member of the hospital's resident staff. Since Robin was going into the army shortly, Denis bought, for £40 ($200.00), his brother's small open-touring Morris. This car was a step up from the Austin, which he'd sold before going to Manchuria.

He found his work in Plymouth agreeable, and after several months had to decide whether or not to renew his contract for another six months. Since he was an earnest Christian, he believed God could speak through Scripture, giving him guidance in a specific way. During his Quiet Time one morning he read from Matthew 2 the passage where Joseph had a dream. An angel warned him to flee with Mary and the Christ child to Egypt. The advice of the angel, **"Be thou there until I bring thee word,"** seemed to be a special message to Denis from God that day. He believed God was telling him to stay on at Plymouth, and not move away. So, that very day, he extended his appointment for another six months.

Denis's hospital duty often included consulting about sick nurses. A new class of student nurses entered the Prince of Wales hospital in April, 1940, among whom was Olive Rogers, whom he was called to see. He learned that soon after her arrival at the hospital she had developed a severely infected smallpox vaccination. Since her father had refused her vaccination in childhood, she had been inoculated only a few days before leaving home as it was compulsory before admission to the School of Nursing. Now, with a severe reaction, Olive had reported to the nursing supervisor, who called Denis, the doctor on duty.

Merely glancing at the festered lesion, he ordered that the attending nurse clean the wound and apply a dressing to the arm. He scarcely noticed the attractive young student, sitting stiffly in her striped blue-and-white uniform. "And hold the dressing in place with an elastoplast bandage," were his parting words as he left the room.

Within 24 hours, Olive reported back to the "sick nurse room," this time with a fiery rash from the elastoplast bandage. "Why in the world did that doctor order the elastoplast?" she complained. "Now I have not only a sore arm, but an itchy one too!" Olive was not too impressed with a treatment which had only compounded her misery.

A couple of weeks later, Denis met Olive again but under different circumstances. She was accompanying a lady doctor to church on Sunday morning, and Denis sat with the two of them during church. After the service the lady doctor mentioned to Denis and Olive, "I must hurry along now, for I'm on duty at the hospital across town."

When she left, Denis turned to Olive and said, "If you're going back to the hospital, I can give you a lift in my car." Olive nodded agreement.

As they drove along in Denis's small Morris, he asked, "How did you learn about this church?"

"During my first week in the hospital, I noticed this lady doctor wearing a 'Crusader badge,' " Olive explained. "I knew that she must be a member of the Christian organization running Bible study classes that I've previously attended. I asked her if such classes were being held in the area. She was very kind to invite me to meet her outside St. Andrew's Church and bring me to the service."

As Denis rounded a corner, he passed several older nurses whom he recognized, walking on the sidewalk. He drew his car up in front of the hospital while Olive stepped out of the car, thanking him for the lift. Then, hesitantly, she apologized, saying, "I'm sorry, but I didn't realize the doctor was expecting to meet and join you at church." Olive's remark passed without his understanding the implication, for he had only chanced to meet the two young ladies.

Several weeks later, Denis was called one evening during supper-break to see a new patient. He was surprised to find Olive the only nurse on duty, since the others had taken off to eat. He asked her, "Could you set up screens around this patient's bed, so I can examine her?" It was a routine request which most doctors gave. "And please bring me an auriscope," Denis ordered.

"A horoscope—?" Olive whispered, her blue eyes wide with surprise.

Realizing the new student nurse's confusion, he smiled and explained gently, "I need the instrument for examining ears."

Olive knew where the ear instruments were kept and promptly produced the auriscope. As Denis left the ward, he casually said, almost as an afterthought, "I'll be finishing my second six-month assignment at the hospital before long. Would you like to go out for a drive with me one day before I leave?"

Olive hesitated. "You have no idea what happened after I rode with you from church to the hospital several weeks ago. A senior member of the nursing staff saw us, and I've been on the mat ever since."

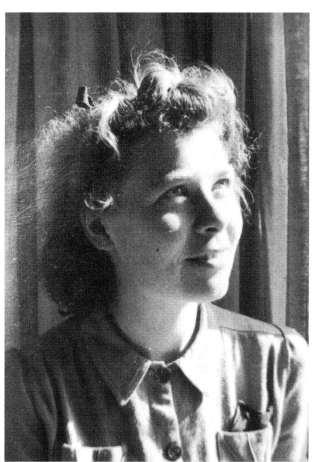

Student nurse, Olive Rogers

25

"Why was that?" Denis looked at her with surprise, saying, "I was merely giving you a lift to the hospital!"

"That's exactly how I explained it!" The color was now rising in Olive's cheeks as she looked down at the tiled floor. She told Denis of her scolding. "My supervisor told me it was most unseemly for me—the most junior nurse in the hospital—to go out socially with a member of the medical staff."

Denis exclaimed it was all foolishness. Romantic ideas had been furthermost from his mind. Olive raised her eyes and looked at Denis' amused face. She decided he might as well know it all. "The nursing supervisor said I'd never complete my training if that was the way I intended to behave. She just wouldn't listen to what I said. The senior nurses have been watching me closely ever since." Olive sighed.

Denis stood looking down at her, almost wanting to laugh. He repeated, "I do wish you'd go for a drive with me."

Surprised at his persistent invitation, Olive said, "There's no way I can be seen again getting into your car."

"That shouldn't be a problem," Denis insisted. "I can simply wait for you in my car on a side road where no one from the hospital walks. Then I'll be careful to drive out away from the hospital where no one will see us." He waited for her decision.

Olive agreed and they decided upon a time. On the designated sunny afternoon, Denis, sitting in his little Morris, saw her walking toward him. He got out of the car, crank in hand, to start the motor with a quick twist, and as the motor responded, ran around to open the car door for her. On their return, as they approached Dartmoor after a pleasant drive, Denis pulled the car over and suggested they go for a walk on the moor.

They walked and chatted until late afternoon, when Denis returned her to the same side street. That was all there was to their brief and impersonal friendship at this time. Actually, Olive was the first girl Denis even had the courage to invite for a car ride. He certainly hadn't considered this a date and soon nearly forgot about it.

He had determined long before that he'd never date or marry any girl, unless she shared his spiritual commitment. He compared the possible perils of a poor marriage partnership to a man or woman standing on a table and taking the hand of the partner on the floor. It would be far more likely for the one on the floor to pull the person off the table, than for the one on the table to pull the partner up onto the table. Therefore, his philosophy was to be most careful in his dating.

Six months passed. Denis had spent the full year at Plymouth and recently moved to his next hospital appointment in the north of England. Christmas was approaching and among the Christmas cards he selected for various friends and relatives was one he had chosen for Olive. Perhaps she wouldn't even remember him, or maybe this lovely girl had caught the eye of some young man. At any rate, he posted the card, wondering whether she would reply.

It was several weeks before he pulled a letter from Olive out of his box. He sat down immediately and answered with a friendly note, telling of his recent hospital experiences. More than a month passed before another letter from her arrived. Again, he answered without hesitation. It was always Olive who delayed writing. Thus, for the next year, their infrequent, platonic correspondence continued.

During this period, Britain became embroiled in war with Germany. The conflict seemed far removed, however, as Denis's appointment in the Yorkshire mining town of Barnsley fully occupied him. On January 18, 1941, he thoughtfully wrote in his diary: "After lunch today I read this passage from *Springs in the Valley*:
> When we want to know God's will there are three things which
> always concur. The inward impulses, the Word of God, and the
> trend of circumstances. God in the heart impelling you forward;
> God in the Book corroborating whatever He says in the heart; and
> God in circumstances, which are always indicative of His will.
> Never start until these three things agree.

Denis finished the notation in his diary by writing: "I feel in my case the three lights are coming in line."

He knew that before long he should put in his application for an assignment in the Colonial Medical Service. On Thursday, January 30, Denis again noted in his diary: "Read from the Bible: 'Get thee out of thy country…unto a land that I will show thee.' (Genesis 12:1). Should I go out as a nonprofessional missionary?"

The next time Denis wrote in his diary was Saturday, February 8th: "Got a letter from Daddy, in which he expressed his willingness and Mummy's for me going abroad. In the evening I read this from *World Dominion*: 'Everyone who leaves the Fatherland for a foreign shore should do so in the character of a missionary; not necessarily preaching his Christianity by his lips, but certainly by his life…. ' "

Everything Denis read these days seemed especially applicable to his present situation. It was as if God, Himself, were speaking to him, assuring him of His leading providences.

On Monday, February 10th, Denis completed filling in his application for the Colonial Medical Service. He had been reading devotional writings accompanied by much prayer, for this was a major life decision. Together with the application, he enclosed a letter explaining that his main motive for applying was his desire "to do God's will," and that he would go in a "missionary spirit." Furthermore, he suggested West Africa as his station of choice. He decided it would be good to have a Christian friend nearby. Cofie George, who had recently married the daughter of a prominent African politician, was now practicing in Ghana.

On Friday, February 21, he received a reply from the Colonial Office. Denis confidently opened the letter, expecting they had duly accepted his application.

However, the letter stated that since he had lost an eye, they wouldn't consider his application.

He couldn't believe it! Simply because of the childhood loss of his right eye they had assumed he would be incapable of filling the rigorous requirements of the Colonial Medical Service. Denis doubted this was the real reason. After all, hadn't he successfully completed three years of surgical training and obtained the F.R.C.S. qualification? The more he thought of his rejection by the Colonial Service, the more he believed it wasn't because of his missing eye, but rather his *stated* Christian commitment.

Why were all his plans thwarted? *Why, Lord, have You permitted this?* He wondered. *Am I unworthy of the honor of working for You? What is the reason for dashing my hopes for this type of medical service?* Denis was despondent, for he had no answers to his questions. What should he do next?

Unbelievably, as though God wanted to comfort Denis in his disappointment, his reading that night from *Springs in the Valley* was just what he needed:

> We cannot expect to learn much of the life of trust without passing
> through hard places. When they come let us not say as Jacob did,
> "All these things are against me." (Genesis 42:36). Let us rather
> climb our hills of difficulty and say, "These are faith's opportuni-
> ties."

The following day, Denis wondered if the Lord might be speaking to him through 1 Kings 12:24, "Ye shall not...fight against...for **this thing is of me**." The verse so impressed him that he took down his Moffatt's Bible translation to read it in another version: "...**for what has happened I have caused to happen**."

However, it was one of his mother's favorite, oft-repeated quotation that encouraged him the most: **"Disappointment—His appointment. Change one letter, now I see."** For the first time, he really understood the saying. But where did God want him? Where was "His appointment?"

3

ARMY AFRICAN ASSIGNMENT

Determined to find God's will, Denis turned his disappointment with the West Africa Colonial Service into action and applied for an appointment in the Sudan Medical Service. *Surely I'll be accepted this time*, he thought, *for I do have good qualifications*. But once again, to his great surprise, he was rejected with the reply: "No vacancies." Since the war had escalated, he now decided it was his patriotic duty to volunteer for the army. Despite his missing right eye, the Royal Army Medical Corps promptly accepted Denis as a lieutenant.

During this time, he and Olive had been corresponding sporadically. *Should I become better acquainted with her?* he wondered. *It's rather difficult to know what she's really like, just writing letters back and forth.* Using a visit to a doctor friend at the Plymouth hospital as an excuse, Denis wrote her that he would shortly be coming for a weekend. His letter also stated he very much hoped she could manage some "off-duty" time to see him.

When Denis got to Plymouth that weekend, the three of them went out for a drive and a walk on the moors. In the evening, a mutual friend invited them home for a meal. There was still no suggestion of any special relationship between Denis and Olive.

However, their correspondence afterward increased with a slowly blossoming, deeper friendship. Denis could manage few leaves to Plymouth from his wartime assignments on the east coast where he was serving in an ambulance corps. Two and a half years passed as the letter-courtship progressed. The threat of being sent overseas pressed Denis into proposing marriage to Olive by letter. "I would love to be officially engaged to you," he wrote. By this time, Olive still had another six months of nurses training. After that, according to her contract, she must spend an additional year of "staffing" as senior ward nurse.

Looking at their calendars, they found a weekend in February 1943 when both were free and agreed to meet at London's Paddington train station. Denis's trip to London was relatively short. His train arrived early in the morning, giving him time to pace up and down the platform until Olive's overnight train reached the station.

After her train pulled slowly into the station, Denis searched the faces of arriving passengers until he spotted trim little Olive. He rushed up to her as the crowds jostled them and the train hissed a cloud of steam. Compartment doors slammed nearby as he rather shyly confirmed the reason for their meeting. "You'll marry me, won't you, darling?"

"For better or for worse!" Olive exclaimed as they embraced.

"Let me take your bag, and we'll go for breakfast here in the station hotel," he suggested. "And let's hope we'll not be interrupted by an air raid siren!" They scarcely noticed the poor quality of the meal as they chatted.

Denis, looking deeply into Olive's eyes, wondered at the providences of God in bringing this lovely Christian woman into his life. "You know, Olive," he said, "I had debated about whether or not to spend the second six-month surgical assignment in Plymouth. While trying to decide, I read in my morning devotional just a few words from Matthew that seemed to speak to me, '...be thou there until I bring thee word.' That made me decide to stay on. And it was during that second six-month period that I met you. Surely God has led us together in a marvelous way!"

"You'd never told me that before," she said, smiling.

Having finished their breakfast, Denis looked at his watch. "It's still early, and it'll be some time before the shops open so we can select a ring for you." He'd planned everything except the discrepancy between the early hour of the train arrivals and the purchase of an engagement ring.

"Never mind. We can walk in St. James Park until the shops open," Olive suggested, easing the situation. So, arm-in-arm, unmindful of the weather that cold, misty February morning, they made multiple circuits of the park. When at last the jewelry shop unlocked its doors, she decided, after lengthy deliberation, on a platinum ring set with a sapphire between two diamonds. Later in the day, they shared their happiness and the rest of their weekend with Olive's father and stepmother, who lived in nearby Reading.

Shortly after their engagement, Denis was transferred to Devon, nearer to Plymouth and Olive. Although they'd known each other for nearly three years, it was a fact that they'd spent relatively little time together. So, whenever his and Olive's schedules permitted, they enjoyed their few hours together, getting better acquainted.

Early in June, both managed to get time off and went to stay with Denis's Aunt May near Poole in Dorset. Denis had something in mind which he realized might shock Olive a bit. As they sat in his aunt's garden overlooking the peaceful harbor, a gentle breeze blew little tufts of Olive's hair over her forehead. He took her hand and asked a question which certainly did surprise her!

"Darling, would you be willing to marry me on my next leave instead of waiting until you finish your hospital commitment?" Denis squeezed her hand tightly and continued to make his point. "You finish your obligation more than a year from now. But I could be going overseas anytime with the war not going well and things so uncertain."

Completely unprepared for this twist, Olive looked at him questioningly. "How can I do it, Denis? You know I have to complete the year's contract with the hospital after my training's finished. It's a requirement."

"I know this is selfish of me, but if I only had you as a wife to come home to—if I just had an image of a loving wife back in England—leaving wouldn't be quite so bad," he persisted. Had he made his point? Did it sound too selfish? He fumbled with a brass button on his officer's uniform.

Olive looked at him hopelessly. Then she looked down, drawing a circle in the sand with the toe of her shoe. After what seemed an eternity to Denis, she finally said, "We must pray earnestly to learn God's will. It isn't an easy decision." They bowed in prayer together.

That evening there was only one topic of discussion, the possibility of an early marriage. It became clear that such an event would hinge first of all upon her passing final nursing examinations scheduled in a few weeks. After that, they would take the next step.

A few weeks later, Denis was assigned to Netley, another army hospital. Because of an unusually large surgeon-exodus to the military, several nearby civilian hospitals in that area invited Denis to do surgery in their facilities. At one of these hospitals, in Wansted, where he was taking calls, he arranged a room for Olive so she could come for a weekend visit. By this time, Olive had passed her examinations. Consequently, on that visit, they decided on a late July wedding when he had a 48-hour leave—that is, if she could make satisfactory arrangements regarding her unfulfilled hospital commitment.

As they talked over the problem and the difficulty it would pose for Olive, Denis only wished he could speak to the nursing matron for her. Of course, this wasn't possible. It would be an anxious time for them both, for not until she found a solution to this matter, could they send out wedding announcements.

The next time they had a weekend together, she told Denis about her approach to the hospital matron. "It wasn't an easy interview," Olive began, "as I still have the year's obligation to the hospital. The matron made me feel very selfish in putting my

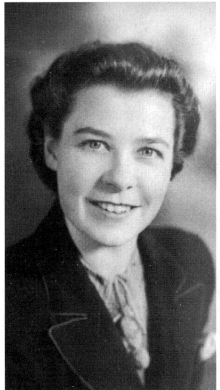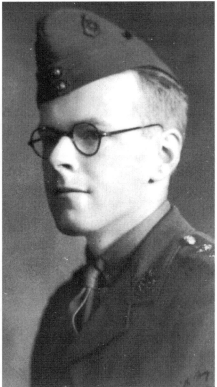

Olive and Denis during their courting days.

personal happiness before the well-being of the hospital patients. She asked me how I could even think of breaking the contract and leaving a year early."

"So how did you convince her?" Denis asked.

"I really didn't," Olive confessed. "After a lot of discussion, the matron finally relented and said I could leave on condition that I paid a sum of money into the hospital coffers."

"I suppose that's only fair," Denis agreed.

Olive drew a long breath. "And so now, after leaving Plymouth, I have only four weeks to prepare for our wedding. But let me tell you about some wonderful things that have happened!"

Denis had been thinking of some practical aspects of the wedding, for with the rationing of nearly everything during the war, he had some questions. "With food rationing and all, how will we plan for the reception? And with clothing rationing, how will——"

"That's what I want to tell you about," she interrupted. "The Lord has really provided. The news of our coming marriage spread around the hospital. When one of my patients, an elderly doctor, learned I was marrying a doctor, he gave me his year's supply of clothing war-ration-coupons. He said, 'I don't need any new clothes. It would give me the greatest pleasure to know you were using these for your wedding gown.' Isn't that remarkable?"

All because you're marrying a doctor," Denis teased.

"But that isn't all!" Olive could hardly wait to tell the rest. "Another student nurse, also planning to be married, had developed tuberculosis and been bedridden several months. When she heard I was getting married, she asked me to come see her. There I stood, masked at her bedside, hardly knowing what to expect. The girl drew a fat envelop from her drawer, saying it would be many months before she could marry. She handed me all the clothing ration-coupons she'd been saving as well as coupons her friends had given her for a trousseau. Can you imagine?"

"How very kind and unselfish. What a loving gesture!" Denis said, overwhelmed.

"Yes, I just couldn't keep back the tears when I said goodbye to her. Here I was going to my wedding while she was going to be in a tuberculosis sanatorium for who knows how long, not really knowing what her outcome might be."

"It truly seems that everything is working out just right." Denis nodded his head in appreciation as he reflected on how their prayers were being answered in such unusual ways.

"With all these coupons, I was able to buy ten yards of white silk taffeta and already have a seamstress friend working on the wedding gown." Olive certainly hadn't wasted any time. She continued, "And she's also sewing up some other dresses—but that's all a surprise. You'll just have to wait!" Now it was her turn to tease. Changing the subject, she said, "But, Denis, you'll never guess what your mother just sent me."

"It would be just like my mother to send you something to show her acceptance of you into the family," he said. "I'm curious to know what it is."

Olive opened her purse, drew out and unwrapped a piece of jewelry. "Have you ever seen this old silver brooch?"

"Isn't that something! That's my mother's favorite brooch, given to her by her mother when she got married." Denis immediately recognized the familiar piece.

Olive opened a second package containing artificial orange blossoms. "And she sent these, which she wore at her wedding. She couldn't have sent anything more meaningful." Olive smiled at her future mother-in-law's sweet gesture.

As the wedding date drew on, Denis realized that his dear parents, whom Olive had never met, would be unable to attend the ceremony because of war travel-restrictions. Nevertheless, there were additional unexpected good things. Somehow, despite wartime sugar rationing, her family was able to procure enough ingredients to make a two-tiered wedding cake, no small feat in 1943!

Olive's white silk taffeta was fashioned into a charming gown and a family friend lent her an embroidered veil. Another hometown friend, an invalid boy whom she had known for many years, made her headdress of white rosebuds and myrtle. And so Denis, in his army officer's uniform, and Olive in her "miracle" gown, were wed on July 28, 1943 in the old Parish Church of Seaford, Sussex.

Their honeymoon, under war conditions, provided an amusing interlude. Denis had booked a hotel room in Iping. Since gas rationing would not allow private car travel, they gathered their bags and left the church by taxi for the railway station. After clambering from the train, they caught a bus to Midhurst. But since there were no seats available on the crowded bus, they stood, hanging on to the bus straps for what seemed like hours. At least Denis now had time to admire Olive's lovely honeymoon dress, which she'd kept secret until she'd changed clothes after the wedding.

Arriving at Midhurst at 9 p.m., they found no taxi service available at that hour and Iping was still three miles distant. They must walk. Undaunted, they transferred necessities for the night into a single small bag, stored the remaining suitcases at the bus station, and set out as daylight was beginning to fade.

On arrival at the hotel an hour later, they presented themselves at the front desk. After thumbing through his reservations' book, the manager said, "I'm sorry, but we weren't expecting you until tomorrow evening."

"That's hard to believe," Denis said, faltering, "could I have possibly confused the date?" He looked helplessly at Olive.

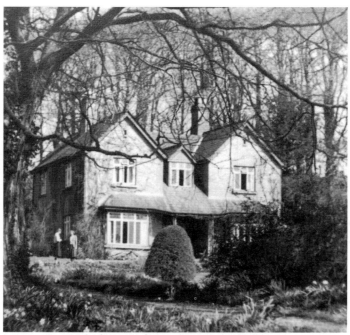

The beauty of Laragh captivated Olive.

The manager quickly sized up the predicament. "Are you newly weds?" he asked. "Yes, we were just married this afternoon," Denis admitted, as Olive nodded.

"Don't worry. I'm sure we can accommodate you with a nice room anyway," the manager said, smiling. "Our dinner service has long-since ended, but I think we could find something for you to eat, also." The hotel did well to scrounge up cold ham and a wilted lettuce salad. But who cared? They were in love and had the next thirty-six hours together.

Iping proved a perfect place for honeymooners. Its wooded paths, edged by wild flowers, invited long walks. The scent of honeysuckle filled the air and encouraged Denis to pick several sprigs which he romantically pressed as a remembrance for both of them. Too soon the honeymoon was over. Denis returned to his hospital and Olive to her parent's home in Reading.

Within days after the wedding, Denis received his overseas posting, which was not surprising, since he had volunteered for overseas duty. The only pleasant feature of the impending assignment was a four week home leave prior to being shipped out. That meant Ireland for Denis. They would go to Laragh, where Olive could meet his folks. He assured her that there was no better place to spend their last weeks together, although she viewed the visit with some apprehension.

Her skepticism was based on a note Gwen Burkitt had written Olive after their engagement: "It appears you have stolen Denis's heart—a very good effort for a young burglar!" Denis laughed when Olive admitted wondering what the lady would be like who had written those words.

Jim Burkitt, on the other hand, had written his prospective daughter-in-law about his own courting days. "Every walk was fairyland when she was by my side." Denis confessed that this was a surprising statement coming from his quiet, undemonstrative father.

When the newlyweds arrived at the Enniskillen railway station, Jim Burkitt met them and warmly welcomed Olive with a sweet smile. He had retired and could now spend his time according to his own wishes. His old corduroy trousers, tweed jacket and a soft gamekeeper's hat were pretty much as Denis had pictured them to Olive, and he was slighter and shorter than Denis, with a balding head.

Olive admitted to Denis later that she hadn't been much impressed with Enniskillen, when they drove in Jim Burkitt's Morris car through the village. It appeared dull and unattractive with its plain gray houses and flat shop fronts. But Laragh was different!

Large beech trees and flowering shrubs of laurel and rhododendron screened the red brick house lying fifty yards or more back from the road. The driveway wound through a well-trimmed lawn bounded by flower beds, Gwen Burkitt's special delight. A tall beech hedge divided the lawn and flower gardens from the barns and sheds, the vegetable garden, and the back drive. Big bow windows on either side of the front porch faced south. Lavender wisteria and climbing pink roses covered the front walls of the house.

"Oh," Olive gasped as she looked around, "how very lovely! Denis, you never described the beauty of your home."

But Denis was looking beyond the familiar surroundings of Laragh for the first glimpse of his mother, who would surely hear the approaching car and come to the front door to meet them. And there she was. Her snow-white hair, caught in a small roll at the back of her head, contrasted with the clear blue of her eyes.

"Welcome to Laragh, Olive dear!" her mother-in-law exclaimed, throwing her arms around the bride. Gwen Burkitt was dressed simply in a plain blouse, tweed skirt and cardigan jacket. Who wouldn't feel immediately at home?

"The flowers—your flowers, I understand, are beautiful!" Olive stood on the front porch looking over the colorful blossoms on every side. "Denis never really described how lovely your grounds are."

"Flowers are *my* hobby. Jim has his birds, but I love the flowers." She would later introduce Olive to some of her rare beauties around the front porch by their Latin names. "Come in, my dear. This is your home too, you know," she exclaimed warmly.

As Olive noticed many pieces of china arranged about the living room, she commented enthusiastically, "What beautiful old English china. Denis told me he upset a cabinet full of china when he was a youngster, but he never mentioned that you collected porcelain."

"Actually, my interest in china goes back to childhood when my mother gave me five shillings to buy a pair of shoes and I returned home with this little Mason's ironstone jug instead of new shoes." Gwen Burkitt held up the small jug which had caught her fancy. Her eyes twinkled as she thought of the amusing incident. "When you and Denis are unpacked and settled, I'd like to take you both around the neighborhood. Everyone wants to meet Denis and his bride."

Before long, she took them from cottage to cottage, where she introduced Olive as "Mrs. Denis." Without exception, faces lit up when they saw Mrs. Burkitt at the door. "Come in, and welcome you are, surely, Mrs. Burkitt. Come in and take a seat." They would invite the three to take chairs by an open turf fire over which large, black cauldrons hung. Gwen Burkitt asked after each member of the families by name. At one home, she removed a tiny baby's garment from her handbag for their newest arrival. It was obvious that everyone loved the thoughtful Mrs. Burkitt.

Olive soon found that her father-in-law was Spartan in all his habits and expected everyone else to follow his frugal example. She smiled when she saw his notice over the bathtub, written out clearly for her to observe:

TWO INCHES OF WATER ARE QUITE SUFFICIENT FOR A BATH.

Wartime restrictions were not new to him, for he had practiced them all his life. Only now he had government backing to make others toe the line too.

How Denis loved showing Olive the various haunts of his happy childhood! A highlight was taking her to Mullaghmore, not to a fisherman's cottage where the family had often gone in the past, but to a small family hotel. The miles of clean strand, the fairy castle on the overlooking hill, the fir-covered mountain trails were all still there as he remembered them, this time to enjoy with his bride.

The idyllic days in Northern Ireland passed quickly, and the return to England and reality came only too soon. Denis and Olive spent their last day together with Olive's folks. They said their farewells at the Reading station, fortunately not knowing the long months of separation which faced them. Neither had they any inkling of the dozens of future farewells that would occur at the same Reading station in years to come.

*****

It was several days before Denis received his final posting. He was to be the officer in charge of a unit, but he had no idea of their ultimate destination. First, a train took his unit to Glasgow, where they boarded a ship. When the troops were issued pith helmets, all assumed they would be heading for the tropics. Denis had sent Olive his military number, which she could use for correspondence, so even on shipboard, her faithful messages began arriving. She had heard "their tune," The *Londonderry Air*, on the wireless. How she missed her Irish lad!

When their ship in convoy with other ships turned east from Spain, Denis knew that the vessel was entering the Mediterranean. He'd met several Christians on the troop ship and soon instigated meetings for Bible study and prayer. It was during one of their Bible study meetings that enemy planes were sighted. Instant orders sounded to go below!

Denis quickly gathered a few belongings, including his Bible and loose notes, and threw them into a bag in case they should have to abandon ship. The fighter planes sunk a destroyer behind them, strafed their deck, killing one, a chap who had been in their study group, and wounding others. Fortunately, this was the closest Denis ever came to seeing active warfare.

Their ship passed through Port Sa'id, the Suez Canal, the Red Sea, Port Tewfik, and finally touched shore at Mombasa in Kenya, East Africa. *There's no place I'd rather be than in Kenya*, thought Denis. He was eager to disembark. He learned that they would be going on to Nairobi. *Uncle Roland made a name for himself as a surgeon in Nairobi, practicing there until 1937*, he recalled. *Although he retired back to England several years ago, I'm sure there are those who'll remember him.*

The ship soon disgorged its human cargo in Mombasa, with the troops boarding a train the same day. In the coastal city the tropical vegetation was a lush green and Denis found the weather hot and humid. But as the train climbed higher through the mountains that evening, the air became pleasant and cool. With the first light of day, as they passed through the flat, grassy game country, he excitedly made out forms of wild animals on all sides of the track—zebras, giraffes, ostriches and gazelles.

On reaching Nairobi, the troops settled into a transit camp while Denis awaited his African assignment. As he had expected, he met several people who had known his Uncle Roland well, including Dr. Gregory, a former medical associate.

This is my opportunity to either disprove or verify the anecdotes I've heard about Uncle Roland for so many years, Denis decided. *I know that he's been a controversial person*. Denis smiled broadly as he spoke with Gregory and inquired about Roland Burkitt.

"As a matter of fact," Gregory admitted, "many in Nairobi are urging me to write Burkitt's biography, since I was more closely associated with him than anyone else." Denis could feel the older man scrutinizing him as he stood before him dressed in his army officer's attire. Finally Gregory said, "I'd guess you were a Burkitt. You have that Burkitt look, somehow. Maybe it's the smile."

Denis didn't mind the comparison, for he had to admit the Burkitts were an unusual family. He had his first question ready to fire at Gregory, "Those stories about his 'cold water treatments' —any truth to them?"

Gregory laughed, saying, "There were so many tales of Dr. Burkitt's drastic treatment of a fever that many of the public feared him. They wouldn't send for the doctor until nearly dead. Nevertheless," Gregory expanded, "Burkitt was greatly respected. For many years he was the only private practitioner in Nairobi, a pioneer in the truest sense of the word. In spite of being highly qualified as a Fellow of the Royal College of Surgeons of Ireland, there was nothing he wouldn't treat. This included animals as well as people!

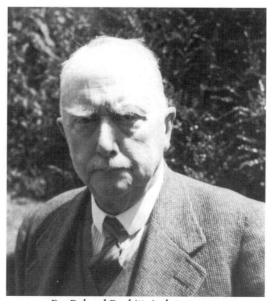

Dr. Roland Burkitt, in later years.

"He was an avid student, always reading the latest in medical literature and putting what he read into practice," Gregory continued, "Very early in his career Dr. Burkitt read in the first chapter of *Wheeler and Jack's Handbook of Medicine* regarding the treatment of fever. The advice was to 'diminish heat production and increase heat loss.'

"He took this advice seriously and from then on advocated cold sponging, cold packs or better yet, cold baths, for all fevers. He always took an oil-sheet with him, frequently pushing the sheet under a bed patient and pouring cold water over him. In spite of opposition and criticism, he carried out what he believed and knew to be right. But this was one of his outstanding characteristics,"

Gregory observed. "He just met criticism with a charming smile."

Denis could picture his uncle as the doctor described him, remembering only too well, years before, his Uncle Roland's determination to do tonsillectomies on him and Robin in their home.

Dr. Gregory illustrated Burkitt's determination with one example of his famous cold water treatment involving a European baby with a high fever. "The mother had bundled the child so it 'wouldn't get pneumonia.' Burkitt stripped off all the baby's clothes, placed it naked in an open work basket which he hung in a doorway to catch a draft. Then he proceeded to douse the baby with cool water from a watering-can. The poor mother was frantic."

Gregory slapped his leg, laughing. "The mother, unable to stand the scene any longer, rushed to a bedroom, locked herself inside, threatening what she would do to the doctor should anything happen to her child. Burkitt took it all calmly, and when the child's temperature came down to normal, he knocked on the door and invited the mother to come out and observe what cool water could do. He didn't leave the house until he obtained her promise to repeat the treatment if the fever recurred."

"So the stories are true!" It was Denis' turn to laugh.

"Not only true," Gregory assured him, "but his treatment worked and was gradually accepted. Many settlers later defended Burkitt's methods and always sent for him as a last resort. He didn't lose a single patient in the terrible Spanish influenza pandemic of 1918, during which he treated Africans as well as Europeans." The doctor, with hands on hips, continued his story.

"Everyone knew about his cold water treatment for fevers. During that flu epidemic, an African family, according to custom, put an old man at the point of death outside their hut to die. They threw a bucket of cold water on him as a final hopeful gesture. Thirty years later, the man was still alive and attributed his good fortune to his relatives using Burkitt's treatment."

"I suppose anyone brave enough to row against the tide is bound to meet ridicule," Denis said with new empathy for his uncle, whom, admittedly, he had previously misunderstood.

Gregory continued in praise of his former associate. He told Denis that Roland Burkitt had published a booklet entitled, *Treatment Of A Fever For Those Remote From A Doctor*, which made his treatment known throughout the whole of East Africa. "Almost every home in Kenya had a copy, costing but a shilling." There was admiration in Gregory's voice, as well as a wry smile on his face. Obviously, he had enjoyed their past association.

Denis broached one further subject carefully, "As a partner, you were in a good position to judge him as a surgeon…."

"Every time Burkitt visited England," Gregory recalled, "he was sure to return with the latest instruments, everything for abdominal work, chest, gynecology, ear nose and throat, orthopedic, even brain surgery. He used only his own instruments, kept in perfect order. Often, during surgery, he liked to recite how he had acquired certain instruments. Usually he'd seen some famous London surgeon using them. As he operated, he would ask for a 'Mr. Walton,' or a 'Mr. Dash,' using the surgeon's names to designate the desired instrument. It seemed," Gregory observed, "that he had every London surgical specialist at his disposal!"

As Denis turned to leave, he thanked Gregory for the insight into his uncle's practice and remarked that he would be looking for his biography someday.

But Gregory had hardly finished. His final words were the best endorsement of all. "Those who worked most intimately with Burkitt would have allowed him to perform any necessary operation on them." He could have paid no greater tribute to Roland Burkitt's surgical skill.

*****

Of his several short assignments in Africa, Denis enjoyed his posting to Gilgil in the highlands of Kenya the most. While there he became acquainted with various missionaries. At one home where he stayed, a wall plaque made a lasting impression:

Only one life, 'twill soon be passed;
Only what's done for Christ will last.

At Gilgil he had his only army leave, just two weeks. How should he spend it? He and a Christian friend decided to go to neighboring Uganda, a providential choice. They traveled by steamer across the wide expanse of Lake Victoria and stopped to see the Mengo Hospital. This institution, he learned, was the oldest mission hospital in East Africa and had been founded by the legendary Sir Albert Cook, who though now elderly, was still residing nearby.

Denis also visited the teaching Mulago Hospital in Kampala, where one day he himself would engage in spectacular research on a childhood cancer. He climbed the foothills of Mt. Ruwenzra (Mount of the Moon), traveled through picturesque Uganda on buses, and stayed with missionaries. On the train back to Gilgil, Denis contemplated, *I'm so thankful for this visit to Uganda. It's convinced me that this is where I should come to work after the war. There are fine Christian missionaries, a lively church, as well as a medical need. Could this be God's* **Appointment?**

What will be Olive's reaction to the idea of coming to Africa? He drew from his pocket a wallet containing pictures of Olive. As he looked at them, he thought, *God led us together, and He has a plan for our lives. We must wait until that plan unfolds.*

Denis's next posting, early in 1945, was to Burma. However his final assignment was to a military hospital in Ceylon. Spending part of the time in an old tuberculosis hospital with little surgery to do, he decided to write an M.D. (Doctor of Medicine degree) thesis for the university at Dublin. He found a local Colombo library, such as it was, adequate for the references he needed for his research. When he completed the project, he considered it "terribly bad," but having nothing to lose, decided to submit it. To his surprise the university accepted it. *Probably*, he thought, *only because I'm a soldier far from university library sources!*

One day, Denis, for the first and only time, "just happened" to be in the servicemen's club when Robin walked in. Robin, who had finished the university with not only a medical degree but also another degree in modern languages and literature, had likewise become an army surgeon. He was passing through Colombo on his way to an assignment in Malaysia. Knowing that Denis was somewhere in the city, he stopped at the club to inquire of his whereabouts. What a joyous reunion it was for the brothers, if only for a few hours!

Shortly after this, and before Denis's next scheduled move to Singapore, the war ended abruptly with the Japanese surrender. Ecstatic, he immediately sent a cable to Olive: FLYING HOME!

This was a bit hasty. For although his trip home was to be by air, it took many flights, each spaced by days or even weeks. His name came up shortly for a flight from Colombo on a Dakota—but only as far as Rangoon. After landing, he immediately put his name on the list for departure. With time on his hands, he bought an eternity ring set with rubies for Olive. Later he went sightseeing with his camera to the city's famous pagoda. That evening, as always, he drew from his pocket his small, well-worn leather picture wallet. He opened it and studied the two photos of Olive. Would she look the same? Now that he was actually on his way home, how he longed to see her!

Time dragged. His next flight took him as far as Calcutta, where he spent three interminable weeks. Wishing to use the time wisely as well as make it pass more quickly, he made ward rounds in a government hospital and observed a smattering of tropical medicine. After flying across India to Karachi in Pakistan, he was again grounded, this time for several days. Would he never reach home? He more frequently than ever took out his billfold and looked at the two pictures of Olive. The next hop was to North Africa, and from there he flew the final leg to Southampton.

As he climbed down from the plane and set his foot solidly on English soil once more, he had only one thought. *Here it is 1946, two-and-a-half years since I've been able to talk to Olive!* He ran to the nearest telephone to call her in East Bourne, where she had been nursing in a hospital during the war.

"I'm coming to East Bourne, darling, and we'll travel together directly to Ireland and Laragh. Nothing will ever separate us again!" Denis vowed.

But he could not look into the future.

4

LOVE FOR OLIVE AND AFRICA

After demobilization from the army in 1946, Denis faced the biggest decision of his life. But it was not a decision he could reach unilaterally, for Olive must share in it equally. What should he do now? Where should he set up his surgical practice? He had seen Africa first hand. He had seen its government hospitals in action and met several wonderful missionaries. Denis felt the Lord was calling him to Uganda. But Olive did not share his dreams. In the privacy of their bedroom at Laragh, they discussed their future.

"I had hoped, Denis, that after being in Africa during the war, your urge to go there and work for the underprivileged would be satisfied." Olive was baring her heart to her husband.

"But Olive, my dear, if you could only see the medical and spiritual needs there!" he urged. "You won't find it all sacrifice either. Africa is a beautiful country. I'm sure you'll love it as I do, once you see the place." Denis was using his best powers of persuasion, painting in her imagination the dark continent's spectacular attractions.

"I'll admit that my ideal is for us to settle in an English village," Olive said. She added with a smile, "But probably that isn't enough of a challenge for you, and your Burkitt blood just has to take you to a foreign land." At last, Olive conceded, saying, "Make your application to the Colonial Office. If they accept your application, I guess we'll go." But perhaps she was remembering his previously turned-down applications for service in West Africa and the Sudan.

"I'll fill out the application today, and we'll see what comes of it." Greatly pleased, with the forms already in hand, Denis set about filling out the papers that very day. He also thought to himself, *After I spent time as an army surgeon in Africa, how can the Colonial Service possibly turn me down again with an excuse over the loss of my right eye?*

In March, a letter from H.M. Colonial Medical Service arrived at Laragh, where they were staying temporarily. The Colonial Service requested that Denis come to London for an interview. It began to look as though an acceptance to government service in Uganda might be forthcoming. Shortly after the interview, the anticipated acceptance letter did arrive, and Olive resigned herself to a life in Africa. It would be an adventure in which they both would share.

April and May were happy days, enjoyed in various pursuits. During the following summer of 1946, they went to Dublin, where Trinity granted Denis his M.D. degree, having previously accepted his memorable thesis, written in Ceylon. They also visited Denis's relatives in Dublin and Cork, but they spent their most pleasurable time bicycling around the picturesque lakes of Killarney. A two-week visit at Laragh by Robin, his wife and five-year-old son, was interspersed with purchasing items unobtainable in Uganda.

A short time later, Denis received another letter from the Colonial Office with an unexpected and disturbing stipulation. "Wives are not allowed to accompany their husbands on new assignments until their work is established."

What a blow, for Olive was now pregnant with their first child! *How can I tell her?* he agonized. *Should I really accept this appointment? How can I leave Olive again after our being together for such a short time? Must I be absent when our first baby is born?*

Denis walked alone up and down the road outside the gates of Laragh, pondering all these questions, wondering what he should do. He knew in his heart he must say, *Yes, Lord, I'll go.* But the struggle went on. This farewell would be even worse than the overseas army departure. When he finally broke the news to Olive, he couldn't blame her for the anguish and disappointment she felt.

"After only six months together, and now we have to face another separation?" Olive couldn't believe what she was hearing.

"There seems to be no alternative." Denis was equally perplexed and down-hearted.

"Why can't you at least delay leaving until after the baby is born?" Olive pleaded.

"I wish that were possible, but the Colonial Service has already set the date for my departure," Denis said with sad finality. Trying to ease her mind, he added, "I'm going to make arrangements with the best obstetrician in Belfast for your prenatal care, and I'll book the nursing home there for your delivery. I think you'll have better care in Belfast than in the Enniskillen Hospital"

They prayed earnestly, and at last Olive bravely decided, "You must go. I'll stay behind, and after the baby's born, I'll join you in Africa." Her acquiescence lifted the burden from Denis, but not the sadness and concern.

Together they began packing their belongings in wooden crates that Denis constructed. They enjoyed looking over their wedding presents, stored at Laragh, and were now finding space in the boxes. When Denis securely nailed the last crate shut, they realized there were far too many boxes for Jim Burkitt's small car to transport from Laragh to the Enniskillen railway station. Denis's father had a practical suggestion—that they hire Willie Jolly and his donkey cart to haul the boxes. Willie was happy to earn a few extra shillings, so they agreed upon a day and hour for him to come with the cart. Denis arranged for some other men to help lift the heavy boxes onto the wagon. However, the cart failed to arrive at the appointed hour. Eventually Willie sent a message that he was unable to catch the donkey. It was the next day before he and the reluctant animal arrived to start the Burkitt goods on its long trip to Africa.

On the day of his departure, September 3, Denis said goodbye to his mother at Laragh while his father took him and Olive to the station for a final farewell. "See you in Africa, my darling," Denis whispered as they clung to each other. His last picture of Olive's sad, stoic face filled his memory for months to come.

After staying briefly with Robin's family outside of London, Denis boarded his ship in Southampton for an uneventful voyage. Not until he reached Mombasa, the port of disembarkation, was he to receive his station assignment in Uganda. As he stood at the ship's rail a few weeks later in the Mombasa harbor, the all-over greenness of the vegetation breathed moisture, adding to the oppressive humidity. Tall palm trees against deep blue skies with billowing thunderheads contrasted with the low red-roofed buildings. It all looked fresh and inviting compared to arid Port Sa'id and the Middle East passed en route.

Government officials met him at the dock and helped him identify his luggage being transferred from the ship to a warehouse. They also took responsibility for putting his crates through customs and loading them on the train. At this point, one of the officials handed him a letter with his assignment:

> DR. DENIS BURKITT IS ASSIGNED TO THE NORTHERN LANGO DISTRICT, AN AREA OF 7,000 SQUARE MILES WITH POPULATION OF 250,000. HE IS TO BE THE DISTRICT MEDICAL OFFICER STATIONED AT THE 100-BED HOSPITAL IN LIRA WITH RESPON-SIBILITIES FOR THE EIGHT OUTLYING SUB-DISPENSARIES IN THE AREA.

Denis spent the night in a Mombasa hotel, and on arising early in the morning, picked up his Bible for his Quiet Time. Walking out into the countryside, away from town, he knew he was in the right place, and that God had called him here. It was the beginning of a new phase of his life. Little did he dream at this time that circumstances would one day lead him into fascinating medical research.

On the two-day train trip to Kampala in Uganda, he shared a compartment with a senior British government official who became so drunk that he had to be carried to bed by the African porters. After they had deposited the gentleman on his narrow bed, he vomited on the floor. *What an example for an "ambassador" of England!* thought Denis. But even this introduction to government service failed to dampen his enthusiasm. Sights, sounds and smells of Africa at every stop and the landscape between, saturated his senses. The sturdy black people, the incomparable beauty of vivid flowering trees set in every shade—from chartreuse to deep forest green—the variety of noble animals, he loved them all!

When his train pulled into Kampala, the superintendent of the Mulago government hospital met him. Dick Drown, the chaplain and head master of the excellent Budo mission school, had also heard of his arrival. Drown had been a "head boy" years before at the Dean Close school in Cheltenham which Denis had attended as a lad. As they renewed their acquaintance, they little realized that the Burkitt and Drown families, in future years, would spend Christmases together in each other's Kampala homes. The following day, Denis met doctors of the Mulago hospital staff, as well as professors in the adjacent college of Makerere Medical School .

But he could not linger in Kampala, for the Lira hospital, 240-miles distant, was in need of its newly-appointed medical officer. An African driver loaded his luggage and that of another new doctor appointee into the open bed of an ancient truck, and the three were off. After about 120 miles, the African driver pulled into Masindi, the destination of the other doctor. Denis noticed the green golf course and the European houses, all very attractive. He spent the night in a Masindi hotel and completed the additional 120 miles to Lira the next day.

Lira's layout was similar to Masindi's with a central golf course and club house surrounded by several well-built homes occupied by eight or so European families. The town itself consisted of a single, unpaved-street, lined by perhaps twenty stores. These were run by Bombay Indian merchants who lived in or near their shops. The Indians were not only the business men, but also the artisans, doing mechanical garage work, carpentry and bricklaying. They owned the only bus company as well. Lira had probably ten times as many Indians as Europeans.

Denis soon learned that the European, Indian and African communities lived entirely separate from each other. However, there seemed to be no racial dislike. Each group had different social backgrounds and therefore didn't associate closely.

The Africans lived in mud-dried brick, or mud-and-wattle, circular or rectangular houses with corrugated iron roofs. These houses were scattered "in the bush" on the periphery of the town. The blacks had no central village community. Instead, their single dwellings usually housed extended families. The women carried water pots on their heads from swamps or water holes along paths which penetrated "the bush" with its shoulder-high elephant grass and interspersed palm trees. Fortunate for them, there were few deadly snakes in Uganda, as Denis soon learned. On the other hand, he found human bites were common and frequently serious, for the Africans often bit each other when fighting.

The African diet consisted mainly of plant foods, as meat was only occasionally available. However, since Lira was less than fifty miles from the Nile, they occasionally had fish. The men folk always ate the few eggs produced by their chickens. Some of the African families kept cows in order to sell milk to the Europeans, but they rarely drank the milk themselves. Uganda, with its plentiful rainfall, had never been a famine area. Most of the local population, Denis learned, were poor, and also illiterate. Better-educated clerks in the hospital had come from Entebbe or Kampala. At this time, mission schools, such as Budo in Kampala, provided nearly all the education available in Uganda.

Denis took up residence the day after his arrival in a large rectangular bungalow with a corrugated iron roof and a veranda all around. It had two bedrooms, and sitting and dining rooms, all identical in size. Outside the back door, a faucet supplied their only running water, fed from a tank which collected rainwater from the roof. Hot water flowed into the bathroom via a pipe leading from an oil drum over a fire outside. The toilet consisted of a wooden box with a hole in it. Under the hole sat a pail which an oxcart driver emptied periodically.

Now why the stipulation about wives not accompanying their husbands? Denis wondered. *I can't see any reason why Olive couldn't have made this trip with me. She could have moved right into our home here. But now I can't really get settled until she arrives and decides how to arrange our goods in the house.*

It was the next day when a young African knocked on Denis's door. "I'm Yusufu. You need a house boy?" Only knowing at this point he desperately needed help in arranging the house, Denis took him on. He specified Yusufu's duties to keep the house clean, make his bed, and go to the market daily for food. However, Yusufu advised Denis, "Bwana, you need cook too. I find one for you."

The following day as Yusufu presented himself garbed in his official senior house boy's "uniform"—a long-sleeved, white gown, loose-hanging from neck to shoes—he also brought several other Africans. It was true, Denis certainly did need a cook. But did he need an assistant cook, an assistant house boy and a gardener as well? He wasn't sure, but feeling sorry for the hopeful crew that Yusufu had collected, he hired them all for what seemed a mere pittance. Soon he learned that all Europeans had this same array of servants.

The hospital at Lira lay across the golf course, about a half mile from Denis's house, so bicycling to work proved quite practical. The medical facility was tin-roofed with open windows. He appreciated, especially during night surgery, that the operating room had been screened to keep out insects and mosquitoes.

His medical staff consisted of one qualified African assistant, Dr. Kunuka, who would later become director of one of the country's larger hospitals. There was also an Indian doctor with lesser qualifications, half way between a medical doctor and a medical assistant. The one European nurse was in charge of the hospital. She had in her home the only refrigerator on the station, since vaccines and other perishable medicines needed to be kept safe. These were subject to vandalism in the hospital. Anyone needing refrigeration, used this one unit.

Besides his routine hospital clinics and surgery, Denis used the hospital ambulance to make monthly rounds at the eight sub-dispensaries scattered over his district. He scheduled one day each week for visiting two of the dispensaries. Trained Africans, who had passed a two-year course in diagnosing and treating simple diseases, ran these units on a daily basis. The African assistants also spent a day or two a week riding out on their bicycles to hold clinics under the trees. They dispensed medicines and screened patients who might need hospitalization at Lira.

Night work, he found, was limited, because patients had difficulty finding their way to the hospital in total darkness. When Denis did have night surgery, he took along his pressure oil lamp and hung it over the operating table. An open-flamed primus stove in one corner of the operating room sterilized instruments in a pan of boiling water. Since the African administering ether anesthetics was merely a trained school boy, Denis usually elected to give spinal anesthetics.

With no adjustable instrument table in the operating room, he became innovative, fashioning a four-sided "box" resembling a wide frame. He slid a reclining patient's legs and hips through the open frame and placed his instruments on a sterile towel on top of the frame-box. His surgical implements, therefore, were handy at the right height regardless of whether the operating table was raised or lowered.

After saving enough money, Denis took a couple of days off for a trip to Kampala. Looking for a car to purchase, he found few

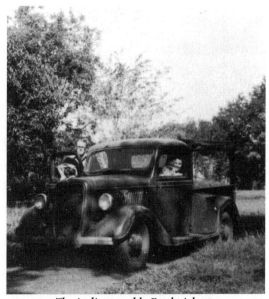

The indispensable Ford pick-up.

cars available in this immediate postwar period. However, as a medical officer, he had received a government priority for the purchase of a vehicle. With this priority document in hand, he bargained for an old Ford pickup truck at £ 140 ($630.00). Its chief drawback was its bad brakes. But since the Lango district was relatively flat and there was practically no traffic, the truck's ability to stop within a hundred feet, he figured, was quite acceptable. He immediately put the truck to use transporting patients between the dispensaries and hospital.

*****

As a surgeon, Denis found a variety of potential surgical cases. Therefore, he was surprised in looking over the operating room log to find previous medical officers had done no more than ten major operations a year. By the end of his first year, he would count up more than 600 operations performed.

He soon found that the most common surgical procedure was for hydroceles (fluid collection around the testicle). He sometimes operated on as many as ten hydroceles a day. The hydroceles were often enormous, containing more than a gallon of fluid. Curious as to their cause, he centrifuged some of the fluid in a test tube, examined the sediment under the microscope, and found it swarming with tiny active larvae of the filarial worm, *Wuchereria bancrofti*. He knew that mosquitoes carried this parasite.

Immediately, Denis became interested in learning the geographical distribution of the disease in his district and plotted its extent by visiting all the medical dispensaries in the area. Usually each African chief could persuade the men in his village to line up naked before Denis for examination. In time, he covered his whole territory, finding about thirty percent of men in the eastern part of Lango district had hydroceles, while only about one percent were afflicted in the western section. He drew his hydrocele data on a map, and later, in 1951, wrote his first paper from Africa, published in *Lancet*, a prestigious British medical journal.

Another disease caused by the filarial worm, elephantiasis, a massive swelling of the leg, also intrigued him. Since the swelling never extended above the knee regardless of the degree of enlargement, he felt the parasite couldn't be blocking lymph channels in the groins as commonly thought. The enormous, "elephant-leg-like" swelling occasionally required amputation of the limb.

Painful, malodorous tropical ulcers, due to fusospirochetal organisms (a spiral-shaped bacteria, together with a rod-shaped bacillus), were also common. Every dispensary had a raised concrete slab for the afflicted patients to sit on while having their ulcers cleaned and dressed. Fortunately, penicillin injections dramatically cured these tropical ulcers. Chronic ulcers of many years' duration often underwent malignant change and required either the excision of the tumors, followed by skin-grafting, or amputation of the leg.

Yaws, another infectious, often multiple, ulcer of the skin, Denis found affected about eighty percent of the surrounding African population. Knowing that yaws ulcers were also penicillin-sensitive and usually cured by a single injection, Denis initiated a plan to eradicate the disease in his district. He requested money for a campaign to control yaws with the intention of giving every man, woman and child a single injection of penicillin to either prevent or cure the disease.

He made all the arrangements for the campaign, but unfortunately it did not materialize until after he left Lira. Subsequently, however, health officers and assistants went throughout the Lango district on their bicycles, armed with penicillin and syringes, and gave injections to tens of thousands of people. Denis learned that the project was highly successful and that yaws disappeared throughout the Lango district. Later, he learned that yaws also disappeared in neighboring districts where there was no campaign at all! Why? No one really knew.

All his patients had chronic malaria and not infrequently some suffered the crippling aftermath of poliomyelitis. Indeed chronic infections of all types were rampant, especially tuberculosis and osteomyelitis (infection of the bone).

*****

The weekly exchange of letters with Olive kept them in touch. He had decided it would be best to warn her that their station was possibly the most unhealthful one in Uganda, since the surrounding country was a flat, low-lying malarial swamp. It was necessary that they faithfully take an antimalarial medication. Perhaps, he decided, if he painted a dismal picture, she would see the beauties of Lira and think it not so bad. Week by week the stack of letters from Olive grew thicker. But he was busy and four months passed quickly.

With the approach of Christmas, he had an opportunity for a first reunion in Africa with his old friend Guy Timmis, who was now a medical officer in Gulu, only seventy miles away. Through Denis's influence, Guy too had decided on the Colonial Medical Service and had actually preceded him to Africa by a few months.

After a pleasant Christmas holiday with Guy, when Denis returned to Lira on December 28, Yusufu handed him a telegram. Hastily, he opened it and read:

DAUGHTER BORN DECEMBER 24. BOTH WELL.
DADDY

He lost no time in wiring his joy to Olive, for the baby was already four days old. Knowing, however, that the baby had not been due for another month, he anxiously awaited a letter from Olive with the details. Had she made it to the Belfast hospital in time? After a week or so, he received her letter from Laragh:

When I saw my doctor in Belfast in early December, he told me not to come again until I came for my confinement. In the intervening weeks the family doctor in Enniskillen could keep an eye on me. So two days before Christmas, I saw the local doctor and he declared all was well. I can hear him saying now, "Go home, Mrs. Burkitt and enjoy your Christmas—the baby's fine—you've got a while to go yet."

That same evening I went into labor. Your dear mother sent for the doctor and at first he refused to come. He said it was probably "a touch of indigestion"—why, he had examined me only that morning—it couldn't possibly be labor pains I was having! Your mother phoned again and again. As the pains increased, he agreed to come at last. One look at me and he said, "I must take her into hospital right away." Your mother wrapped me in her fur coat. Molly [the maid] packed my suitcase and off we went into that dark December night, with freezing fog. The wind-screen wipers on his car were not able to cope with the weather and the poor doctor had to repeatedly stop and get out and scrape the frozen fog away before we could proceed. The five miles to the hospital seemed like fifty!

I'm sure the doctor felt rather humiliated. And so after all the loving arrangements you made, Denis, I was taken into the dreaded local hospital and my Belfast plans went by the board. Judith Marion Burkitt was born early the next morning, 24th December. I looked out of my hospital room and saw the bare branches of a tree rimmed in frost, sparkling like diamonds and thanked God for the precious jewel he had given me in our newly born daughter....

My darling Olive, and little Judy. How I wish I'd been there, but I'm thankful all went well, and now you'll soon be with me. Denis drew a long sigh, slowly folded the letter and added it to the pile. In her next letter, Olive said she had contacted the Colonial Office for passage to East Africa and February 21 was her sailing date. The ship was due to arrive in Mombasa on the 10th of March .

*****

March arrived, and the date for Olive's ship to dock in Mombasa was imminent. In anticipation, Denis drove his truck to Tororo on the Uganda-Kenya border. There he caught the train for the rest of the journey to Kenya's port city. He was pleased to find Dr. Hugh Trowell, a professor from Makerere Medical School, occupying the same coach with him on the train. They had met at the Mulago hospital when Denis first arrived in Kampala six months earlier. Now they had much to talk about,

"When did you first come to Africa, Hugh?" Denis asked, little realizing, as he opened the conversation, what impact this man would have in different periods of his life.

"My wife and I came out in 1929, shortly after I graduated from St. Thomas's in London." Trowell's face radiated a pleasant smile.

"I understand that you were the first to describe Kwashiorkor (a severe nutritional deficiency in children). Tell me about it," Denis said as he settled in his train seat, prepared for a long discussion.

"I was working in Kenya in the early years, in Mombasa and Nairobi," Hugh said, crossing his legs. "I kept seeing malnourished children with the same findings—protruding abdomens, a reddish coloring of the skin and hair, edema (swelling) of the legs, a peculiar skin rash and severe diarrhea with undigested food in their stools."

Hugh drummed his fingers on the armrest of his seat as he recalled how many of these children had died. "I'd never seen anything like it described in medical textbooks and figured it was probably a vitamin and protein deficiency. Believe it or not, this disease in Uganda was being diagnosed as congenital syphilis. I began compiling findings on these children from many medical records and finally published the results."

"Wasn't there a lady doctor working simultaneously on the same problem elsewhere, Hugh, unknown to you?" Denis interrupted.

"That's right," he admitted. "While I was investigating the disease in East Africa, Dr. Cecily Williams was observing the same symptoms in children in West Africa. Her first report in 1931 attracted some attention to the disease in Britain."

"Did you two ever meet and discuss your findings?"

Hugh smiled. "Yes, we finally met in 1945 after the war and had some interesting discussions. In fact, I told her that from then on, I too would refer to the disease as 'kwashiorkor,' as she'd given the disease this name from its African designation in her area." Hugh continued somewhat hesitantly, "My continuing interest in this illness and other nutritional problems, however, bothers some of my colleagues at the Makerere medical school. They think that food studies have become an obsession with me." Hugh laughed. "Maybe they're right. Nutrition has always been a special interest of mine. In fact, right now I'm headed for Nairobi to do a dietary study."

"How's that?" Denis had become interested in this self-effacing man with an investigative bent.

Trowell pulled a letter from his shirt pocket saying, "The officers of the East African Railway have requested I do a nutritional survey on their workers in Nairobi. They're questioning if their diets are adequate."

"So there are those who appreciate your work and consider your expertise valid in nutritional matters," Denis said. He empathized with this doctor whose medical compatriots failed to appreciate his bent to nutritional research. He thought, *Here is a man who labors quietly and carefully, making important findings in the nutritional field, but his colleagues scoff at his work!*

✳✳✳✳✳

With sweat streaming down his sunburnt face, Denis stood on Mombasa's wharf two days later, scanning the passengers who crowded the rail of a docking ship. At last he spotted Olive, holding up baby Judy for his first glimpse of their little daughter. What a thrill! He could hardly keep back the tears. Oh, how he'd missed his dear Olive, and now at last she was actually to be with him in Africa. As she walked down the gangplank, he waited on the dock ready to embrace her and take his own dear little baby in his arms.

"Welcome to Africa. How was the voyage, dear?" Denis kissed his wife and their sweet baby, finding it difficult to believe they had actually arrived.

"I'm so relieved to be here," Olive explained, "you'll never know how worried I was on shipboard. Six children in our cabin came down with not only the measles, but mumps and chicken pox as well! I was worried the whole way over that the baby would also get sick!" At this point, Olive wasn't even minding the humidity, heat, or confusion on the wharf.

"You'd better take some of these clothes off the baby—she'll be getting prickly heat," he said, noticing the baby's warm clothing and handing Judy back to his wife. "Remember, you're in the tropics now."

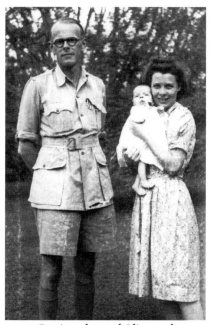

Denis welcomed Olive and Judy to Africa.

Olive laughed, saying, "Before we left England, dear sister Lucy made Judy this beautiful pink silk dress and knit her this wool cardigan for her to wear when we landed in Mombasa. She's dressed especially for you, Denis!" Olive began stripping the hot clothes from the baby, and laughed again, "Neither Lucy nor I realized how inappropriate these fine clothes would be!"

"I've booked rooms in a nice little hotel for a few days so you can rest before we go to Uganda," Denis informed her, for he knew that the long voyage had been tiring. "This will acclimate you a bit before we leave for Lira."

"How thoughtful, Denis dear! It'll be nice just to stand and sit where there's no movement," Olive said. "And I'd like to change my own heavy clothes. I had several summer frocks sewn during the dead of winter in Enniskillen and wondered at the time if I'd ever be warm enough to wear them."

Several days later on the train to Kampala, Denis prayed silently that Olive would learn quickly to love Africa as he did. It wasn't long before she exclaimed, "Denis, you never told me how beautiful the African skies are—such a deep blue, and the cloud formations are so bold and unusual!" And a bit later as the train gained altitude and the scenery changed, she smiled and said, "You never told me about the beautiful eucalyptus trees, the gorgeous bougainvillea, all this green foliage—and back at the hotel, those white, waxy frangipanis with the delicious peach-like fragrance…"

"But I did tell you about the animals we're going to see from the train tomorrow as it passes through the game parks." Denis had a feeling that it really wasn't going to be long before Olive too loved Africa.

He was right, for she excitedly pointed through the train window as the sun broke through the morning mists over the great plains, "Look, a giraffe! I can just see it through the mist—and there's a whole herd of zebras. This is so beautiful and far-removed from the ugly war ruins in England. It seems unreal." Those were the words Denis was waiting to hear.

"The country isn't so bad," Olive told him as they loaded her luggage in the back of his pickup. "But your truck! I'm not so sure it's a step up from your little Morris!" she joked. It took her a while to get used to the undependable brakes. Upon their final arrival in Lira,

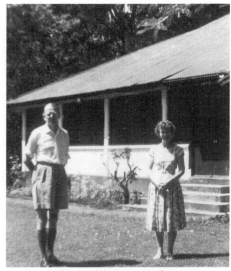

The Burkitts pose in front of their Lira home.

even Denis began to see the *boma* (European community) in a different light, through Olive's eyes. "With those lovely flowering tropical trees, it's like living on the edge of a park," she exclaimed. And yes, their house was spacious and quite adequate. "But the servants," she gasped, "Denis, you never told me that we have six servants!"

"Didn't I? Well, I suppose I forgot to mention them," he replied, almost sheepishly. "I did have five servants, but just arranged for an ayah to help you take care of the baby. I hope you're not disappointed."

"Here I thought I was going to have to do everything about the house myself, including cooking, shopping, washing nappies—everything!" Olive's eyes shone with joy and appreciation. "This is marvelous. But I mustn't get spoiled." Yusufu and the other servants breathed easier as well, for they knew that they would enjoy working for the *bwana's* wife.

What made Denis especially pleased was that Olive soon enjoyed going on the safaris around the district with him. Yusufu had the cook prepare food for the trips while he packed beds and mosquito nets and came along to set everything in order. The Africans had never seen a white baby and came for miles just to see little Judy.

Sometimes, as they returned to Lira in the dark after a busy day, bumps in the road caused the headlights to go on and off and added excitement to the trip. Gaps in the truck's floor boards allowed dust to pour through from the dry roads. During rains, dirty water splashed in. But Olive was a good sport. "Things are washable," she'd always say.

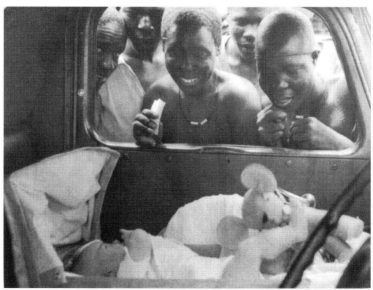

Judy waves and the Africans admire.

When Denis first arrived at Lira, he had become acquainted with a missionary couple, Alf and Gladys Peaston, whose mission station at Boroboro was only four miles away. After Olive and Judy had joined him, the families became even closer and Gladys was like a mother to Olive. Every Sunday afternoon, Denis and Olive went out to Boroboro for a little service, followed by supper with the Peastons, or Alf and Gladys came to Lira to be with the Burkitts. Since their government neighbors had other interests, Denis and Olive particularly enjoyed this Christian fellowship. Occasionally Alf accompanied Denis on overnight safaris in his district when Olive couldn't go along.

Life at Lira was pleasant. Even though not living in luxury, Denis and Olive were together as a family, and in their very first home. He could slip away from the hospital each noon for lunch with her, and they were also able to spend time together in the evening reading books, or just sitting out on the veranda behind insect-proof netting.

At times they'd watch an approaching tropical rain with fascination. The spectacular African sky would suddenly become black in the distance, and as the storm moved rapidly toward them, the edge of it enveloped the remaining blue sky. They would estimate at just what moment they should flee indoors as torrents of rain suddenly poured in loud crescendo on their iron roof like erupting kettle drums in a grand symphonic finale. In a half-hour or so, the storm would pass over and the sunshine brighten the refreshed landscape once more.

*****

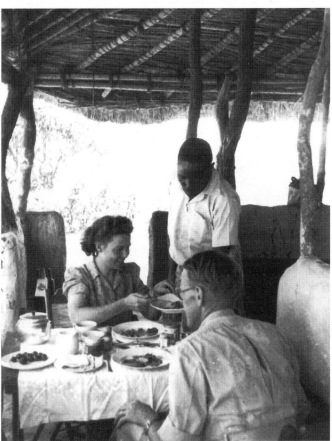

Yusufu serves dinner on a district safari.

56

Denis, at this time, was one of only two qualified surgeons for all of Uganda's 6,000,000 people. The more Olive thought about this, the more she began resenting his assignment to this remote outpost. Finally she spoke out, "Do you know what your mother said to me before I left home? I guess she knows you pretty well." Olive laughed. "She said, 'Don't let Denis be too much of a doormat, dear.' "

"Mummy said that?" Denis grinned. "I do try to follow orders."

"Yes, but is this your reward for never questioning and always accepting what comes because of your devotion to your calling? Really, Denis, with your qualifications, the M.D. and fellowship in the Royal College of Surgeons, it seems that you deserve to be at the teaching hospital, not wasting your talents out here in the district." There! Olive had said aloud what had been on her mind for some time.

"I suppose you have a point, dear." Denis could see advantages in a different assignment. "I could be doing more refined surgery of various kinds in Kampala. I'd have better instruments and certainly a better operating room." However, the longer he worked in Lira, the more he daily thanked the Lord for the experiences he was having. Since there was no one with whom to consult on difficult cases, he had had to become self-reliant and able to make quick decisions. *Yes*, he decided, *Lira is a training and proving ground for me. It's exactly what I need—to serve my "apprenticeship" 240 miles by dirt road from the nearest x-ray machine.*

Denis had worked in Lira just eighteen months when he received a telegram that would change their immediate and future lives completely. Olive had her wish. The telegram read:

> IAN MCADAM SICK. YOU ARE HEREBY TRANSFERRED TO THE DEPARTMENT OF SURGERY, MULAGO HOSPITAL, KAMPALA. URGENT.

5

EARLY YEARS IN KAMPALA

Soggy jungles, mosquito-swarming swamps, parched deserts and exhausting mountains did not diminish the determination of twelve foot-weary but resolute young missionaries. Neither did weakening bouts of dysentery or threats from wild animals and hostile natives stop the brave band from Mombasa who finally ended their *800-mile expedition* at their goal in Uganda. Here was the place to start a medical work with the hope of eventually winning Africans to Christianity. The year was 1896.

The group was unusual in that among its number were three women. One, Katherine Timpson, would later become the wife of the company's young doctor, Albert Ruskin Cook.

Dr. Cook was soon seeing patients and operating in a rude hut with a mud floor. He built additional huts as necessary to accommodate his growing number of needy patients. Finally, he erected the fifty-bed Mengo Hospital, said at that time to be "the finest building in all of Uganda." Cook not only served the Africans in his hospital, he also traveled to outlying villages on his dilapidated bicycle. Katherine usually accompanied and assisted her husband. Her mode of transportation was a mule. On one such two-month trip, they saw over 5,000 patients and did twenty major operations!

During World War I, the Cooks, with their medical assistants, dealt with four epidemics simultaneously: spinal meningitis, cholera, smallpox and bubonic plague. Nearby Mulago Hospital was to become an outgrowth of Cook's syphilis clinic, which had answered the need for treatment of this disease in a deadly epidemic of former years. Both the doctor and his wife suffered periodically from recurring bouts of malaria. Katherine died of cerebral malaria in 1938. Sir Albert Cook was still living when the Burkitts moved to Kampala in 1948, but in his retirement, because of old age and ill health, made few public appearances. Dr. Hugh Trowell was serving as Cook's physician during his declining years.

It was to this medically historic city of Kampala, embracing both the outlying Christian Mengo hospital and the government Mulago facility, that Denis was called. No sooner did Denis and Olive arrive at Mulago Hospital than surgical patients inundated him from morning to night. The chief surgeon, Mr. Ian McAdam (British surgeons are given the title of "Mr."), had become partially incapacitated by a peptic ulcer. For a time he turned over much of his surgery to Denis.

In 1948, this government hospital had 400 beds and was also the teaching institution for Makerere Medical School, the only college training African doctors for Kenya, Tanzania, Zanzibar and Uganda. Makerere was still small, taking only about fifteen new students a year. Later it would become affiliated with London University, which sent out external examiners each year to ensure that graduating students were up to British standards. Medical students in 1948, however, had only to finish secondary school (equivalent to high school) before beginning the five-year curriculum at Makerere. Realizing the rare privilege they had for education, the African students were diligent, rarely taking time for recreation.

Perched on one of several flat-topped hills surrounding Kampala, Mulago Hospital itself consisted mainly of many single-storied, brick buildings with corrugated roofs, connected by covered walkways. These buildings housed, in separate

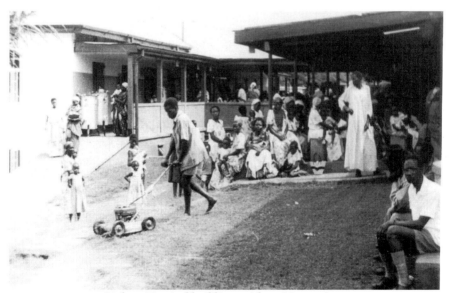

Mulago Hospital buildings with waiting patients.

wards, the various medical services—surgery, obstetrics and gynecology, pediatrics, internal medicine, and orthopedics. Although it was far-better equipped than the Lira Hospital, Denis still considered the buildings primitive, compared to those in England.

All the doctors working in the hospital lived in bungalows on Mulago Hill near the medical facility. Denis could again lunch at home, or if called out for a night emergency, arrive on the ward in a matter of minutes.

Mulago hospital, on the edge of Uganda's capital city, Kampala, was about two miles from the city center. In the late 1940s the city's population stood at 40,000 and had no high-rise features. Its buildings were a mixture of modern, several-story-high structures and one-story Indian open-fronted dukas. A red-brick Protestant cathedral, a Roman Catholic cathedral, the University of Makerere, and an Islamic mosque dominated other flat-topped hills surrounding Kampala. The well-planned city itself boasted broad, well-drained streets and residential avenues lined by lavender jacaranda, yellow acacia and bright orange flame trees. Its many unoccupied areas, at this time, presented a park-like atmosphere.

Denis was pleased that Olive immediately liked Kampala even better than Lira, for there were good shops where one could buy nearly anything desired. She shortly made many new friends, not only among the Europeans but also among educated African and Asian families, and she became a member of the Uganda Council of

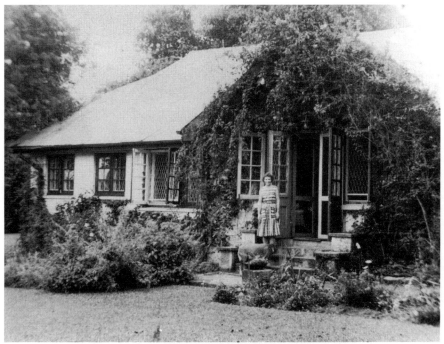

Olive stands on the front steps of the Burkitt bungalow.

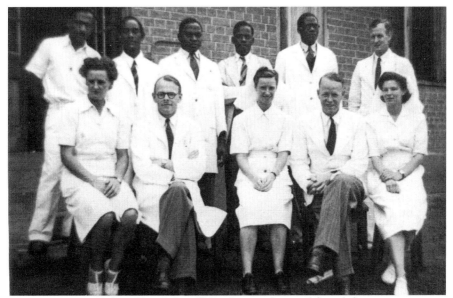

Mulago Hospital staff. Denis seated second from left;
Ian McAdam seated second from right.

Women. This organization of all races and creeds sought to advance the status of the country's women. Kampala offered occasional concerts, a Uganda Society with meetings and scientific publications, and a good school for children up to age twelve.

Creeping vines covered their new house, which had three bedrooms, living and dining rooms, an office for Denis, an inside pantry and outside kitchen, a bathroom with hot and cold water and an actual toilet, electric lights, and a telephone. Of course, they had brought Yusufu with them, but not the other servants. Since Olive had an electric stove, she decided to do her own cooking. Yusufu and the children's ayah, who also did the laundry, occupied the servants' rooms.

Denis was pleased to have not only his own workshop but also a garage for their first new car, a comfortable Chevrolet sedan. They purchased the car for £ 600 ($2700.00) shortly before leaving Lira. To Olive's special delight, a terraced garden had mango and avocado trees as well as many brightly-colored flowering shrubs. She tended its fragrant rose bushes and English summer annuals herself.

Mr. Ian McAdam, though younger than Denis, had enviable qualities of leadership, being a superb surgeon and administrator. He was athletic, and served as captain of the Ugandan tennis team, captain of the Ugandan cricket team, and captain of the Ugandan golf team. Besides this, Denis observed, he was good-looking and a hard worker. Although Ian himself never wrote scientific papers, he encouraged other doctors to do so. He was an excellent teacher, and Denis was not surprised when he was elected senior surgeon at the medical school.

Olive looked at things a little differently. With wifely loyalty she felt Denis deserved to be the senior surgeon. Ian was not only younger than Denis, but had received his fellowship in the Royal College of Surgeons later as well. "Why didn't they appoint you as senior surgeon at Makerere instead, Denis?"

With not only an honest evaluation of reality but also personal humility, Denis put Olive's evaluation to rest. "I couldn't be working with a finer man. Ian is so good at everything, I just can't feel jealous of him. He's much better suited for this job than I would be." In time, as Olive became better acquainted with McAdam and his family next door, she decided that Denis's judgment had certainly been right.

At Lira, Denis had always worn khaki shorts, knee-length stockings, and a khaki bush jacket. But very quickly Ian, as chief, suggested that all doctors wear white coats over a white shirt to add dignity. So the doctors all went to town and had clinical coats tailored at an Indian shop. Usually the Africans, upon promotion, immediately donned long trousers, feeling that wearing shorts was beneath them. Thus, within another year, the European doctors mutually decided it would be appropriate if they too wore long trousers.

Denis and Ian had separate surgical wards with assigned residents in training. Each Tuesday, they listed on a blackboard all the patients needing surgery that week and decided between them the assignment of cases. Before long another capable surgeon from England, Mr. John Croot, joined the staff. The university appointed

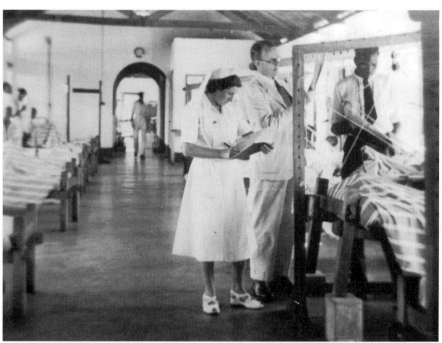

Denis making rounds with resident on the orthopedic ward.

him as its first Professor of Surgery. As the doctors walked between the wards, Denis always felt more comfortable walking with the residents behind the other two surgeons.

Shortly after they settled in Kampala in 1948, Denis received an unexpected phone call. Jack Darling, whom he hadn't seen since their meeting at an Intervarsity Fellowship conference in Ireland when they were both medical students, was in town at a hotel. Denis insisted he stay in their home instead. Now also a surgeon in the Colonial Service, Jack's assignment was in a Tanzanian hospital. At the suggestion of his chief medical officer, he had come to Kampala to learn the type of problems he would be facing in East Africa.

Denis took him around the hospital and medical school, introducing him to his colleagues. During his short stay, Jack learned valuable information on the treatment of various tropical diseases which were all new to him. While at the Mulago Hospital, he attended a staff meeting where Denis presented a paper on hydroceles, based on his experiences in Lira. About a decade later, Darling would himself join the Mulago staff in the surgery department.

*****

Years before, when Denis had visited the nearby Mengo Mission Hospital during army leave time, he never dreamed that a second daughter would be born in this famous institution. Carolyn was born on January 30, 1949, about a year after their move to Kampala. While in the hospital, Olive learned more of the fascinating history of Mengo, East Africa's first mission hospital, dating back more than fifty years. After hearing exciting recitations concerning the Cooks' medical work, Olive had to admit, "Denis, we're so privileged to work in the very same district of Africa!"

Soon baby Carolyn had a new name. The African servants, unable to pronounce "Carolyn," called her "Casolina," and from this, the family derived the nickname, "Cassy."

About the time when Denis transferred to the Mulago Hospital, Guy Timmis also shifted to Kampala. This move became crucial for Guy, as he shortly fell in love with an Australian nurse, Dawn Brewer, who worked at the Mengo Hospital. Being a shy person, even after months of friendship, Guy progressed slowly with his courtship. Since he and Dawn were both in their late thirties, in all fairness to the lady, the medical superintendent of Mengo felt that Guy should not prolong the friendship unless he was serious. Therefore, the superintendent actually came and spoke to Denis and Olive of his concern for Dawn, knowing they were Guy's best friends.

Olive decided to help their bashful friend in his pursuit. Her opportunity came when he dropped by their home before escorting a patient to Nairobi for treatment.

In an offhand way, half jokingly, she said, "Guy, what about coming back with an engagement ring since there are better jewelers in Nairobi than in Kampala?"

He smiled, blushing a bit and said, "Do you think so?" He did take the hint and returned with the ring. Guy and Dawn were married a few months later, with Denis acting as best-man at the wedding.

*****

The longer Denis worked at Mulago, the more he became aware of the large number of patients with crippling diseases. He kept seeing patients with poliomyelitis, tropical ulcer with cancer, elephantiasis, (all needing amputation), and various injuries incurring loss of a limb. Looking at the unfortunate patients, unable to get around or support themselves except by begging, he wondered how he could help them and determined to find a solution to their sad dilemma. Since his first home leave to England was due shortly in 1949, Denis decided to use the vacation time taking an orthopedic course. To do this, he would have to extend their leave to five months.

The whole family viewed with excitement the upcoming furlough, for they especially looked forward to their stay at Laragh. Little Judy, now three years old, viewed Laragh as a fairyland from all her mother's stories. And Olive had not exaggerated, for on their arrival at Laragh, Gwen Burkitt's flowers were more beautiful than ever. Denis quietly observed an interesting new side to his undemonstrative father, who immediately fell in love with his tiny granddaughter, Judy.

"Judy, my girl, have you seen Alice this morning?" he would ask the wide-eyed little girl.

"No, grandpa, where is she?"

"I'll bet if we go down to the Echo House, we'll find her there." Delight etched Jim Burkitt's face as he used his imagination, rarely before seen. The "Echo House" was a shed in a back field, newly named for the game. "Why don't we go and find her?"

And with that, the two would leave the house hand in hand. Judy later returned to repeat all kinds of stories which her grandfather had concocted about "Alice." But he also taught her about his birds.

"Listen to that bird call, Judy. Do you hear it? Now if you look closely, you can see it sitting on the low limb of that tree. Do you see it?" Patiently he would try to identify bird songs for the child, as well as to point out, through his binoculars, various of his feathered friends.

Granny couldn't hear enough stories about their African experience. She and Olive visited and did needlepoint while sitting in the drawing room's window-seat facing west toward the copper beech tree in the yard. Here, as the shadows of the long summer evenings lengthened across the lawn, the setting sun filtered its light through the branches and leaves of the beech. The warm glow of being home again permeated the room as the women chatted and Denis and his father read books or magazines.

"I'm going up to London next week, you know, Daddy. My orthopedic course begins then," Denis reminded his father. "I hope you don't mind if I leave the family here with you and Mummy." He knew his parents would relish the idea. In fact, his mother had previously requested that the family stay with them at Laragh. This was a fairyland indeed for Olive as well as Judy. She loved Denis's mother and actually preferred staying in Laragh to visiting her own father and stepmother in England.

The home leave passed too quickly for everyone, and the family's return to Uganda became imminent. Denis had made good use of his time, acquiring many practical ideas he wanted to put to use. He was anticipating how he could make cheap, practical leg prostheses for his crippled African patients.

After their return to Uganda, it was not long before his newest hobby was fashioning artificial legs. He had learned in London about malleable plastic used in airplane construction. This he considered suitable for leg prostheses. He devised an artificial limb by covering with the malleable plastic a length of pole equivalent to the portion of an amputated leg. After making a plaster of Paris cast of the leg stump, he molded the end of the prosthetic leg to fit neatly over the stump. He shod the "foot" with a piece of durable tire rubber. Such an artificial leg could be made for about £ 1 each ($4.00) and could last from five to ten years, depending on its use. He began fitting many appreciative patients with new limbs.

Denis also contrived leg braces for polio patients out of rebars (long metal bars) ordinarily used in concrete construction. Acquiring these free from the public works department yard, he formed "caliper" braces with the metal rods attached to the boot heels. Children's shoes were made with no toe caps so that as a child grew his toes could protrude and the brace be fitted lower on the leg. Thinking of everything, he arranged for the local Salvation Army hostel to accommodate the patients while they were being fitted for braces. Before long, Denis published another medical report on his innovative, cheap prostheses and braces.

From this inauspicious beginning, the prosthesis industry grew and later became a full-time orthopedic department. African trainees from other countries than Uganda learned to fit and make the braces, while these and the artificial limbs became increasingly more sophisticated.

*****

Many of Denis's colleagues on the Makerere University teaching staff, like he himself, had gone to Africa at God's calling, having chosen remuneration from university or government services instead of from missionary societies. These Christian doctors felt a spiritual responsibility to their patients. However, there were problems in communication, since the Africans in Kampala represented eight different language groups. The doctors solved the language barrier when they formed a team and undertook the hiring of a full-time African, Pastor Galiwango, to minister as a chaplain in the hospital. Pastor Galiwango's salary, house, office, literature for distribution, as well as a small car, were all provided by the physicians..

The doctors also set up a hospital broadcasting system with headphones in every ward. A notice, announcing sermons by the various physicians, distributed before a Sunday's service, assured an audience. Since the patients had confidence in their doctors, they faithfully listened to the messages translated into various languages by Pastor Galiwango.

Some of the doctors, including Denis, had an active outreach program as well, going to the local prison, to hold Bible studies with the inmates. During this time, Denis became a lay preacher in the Anglican church, with speaking assignments every month or six weeks.

*****

One day in 1950, a tall, well-built European addressed Denis outside the hospital conference room, "Dr. Burkitt.?" he

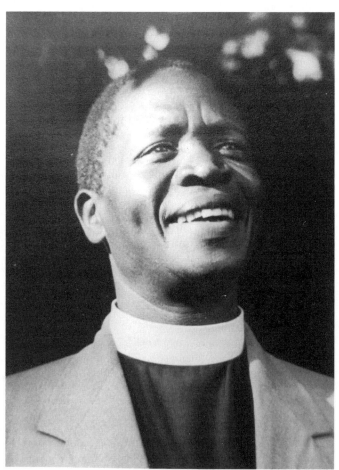

Mulago Hospital's chaplain, Pastor Galiwango.

asked, then added with a chuckle, "I'm sure you're a Burkitt—you look like one! I was told you were in Kampala. I'm Ted Williams."

"You're right. I am Burkitt," Denis replied. "Ted Williams—you're a doctor from northern Uganda. I've heard of you."

"I'm from the Kuluva Hospital up north," Ted responded. As they chatted, he explained his instantaneous recognition of Denis as a Burkitt. "I was born in Nairobi. My father was chief engineer in the Kenya Survey Department and knew your uncle, Dr. Roland Burkitt, quite well. Your cousin, William Burkitt, is a friend of mine. There's a strong family resemblance!"

"Others have said the same," Denis replied. "I hear you have quite a unique hospital at Kuluva that you pioneered yourself."

"You'll have to come up and see it," Ted invited, pulling from his pocket a pen and a scrap of paper. He not only invited the Burkitt family to come for a visit, but drew a crude map with directions showing how to reach his mission hospital.

"Why don't you come on over for lunch and meet my wife, and we can talk more about it," Denis suggested. This was the beginning of a lifetime friendship, as the two men and their families became acquainted. Not only Ted, but also his younger brother Peter, had been born in Nairobi. As young men, both had gone to England for their university and medical education. Ted finished several years before Peter and married a proficient English surgical nurse, Muriel. As newlyweds in 1941, they decided to begin their medical missionary work in remote Arua, a desperately needy area of Northern Uganda.

After several years, the Williams expanded their medical practice, including leprosy work, at a new 200-acre site, Kuluva. In this area, only seven miles from Arua, 20,000 people had no medical help. Ted made sun-dried, mud bricks and constructed both their home and multiple, small hospital buildings. He dammed up a stream from the river and fashioned a serviceable water supply. In 1948, Peter, later to become an ophthalmologist, joined Ted and Muriel. Ted's and Peter's retired parents also joined them that year. It took the combined hard work of all five of them to build up the new institution.

Not long after their first meeting with Ted, the Burkitts decided to make the trip in their Chevrolet to visit the Williams in Kuluva. The trip took them through Masindi, where Denis had spent his first night in Uganda between Kampala and Lira. En route, they passed by the awe-inspiring Murchison Falls. Lingering a bit in the Murchison National Park, they admired its wild elephant herds, impala deer, long-legged birds and vast array of protected animals. At Pakwach on the Nile, they crossed by ferry into the West Nile District of Uganda. Finally, they pressed on through cool wooded terrain another eighty miles to Kuluva. It was quite a trip!

As Denis was being shown around the hospital grounds after their arrival, he spoke with great admiration, "This is quite a layout, Ted! You built all of this?"

"It took us about five years, and we're still adding to it gradually, but the buildings are simple, made of mud-dried bricks, about a half million at least! African workmen that we've trained now do most of the building." As he spoke, Ted moved his arm in an arc encompassing about forty small buildings. "These," he explained, "are occupied by our three hundred in-residence leprosy patients who are receiving courses of intensive treatment. Over there is our thirty-bed hospital, where we see about fifty thousand outpatients a year."

Denis could see that Ted enjoyed the mechanical aspects of his work as well as the medical, for the Williams menfolk kept all the electrical equipment at the hospital in repair. Ted readily admitted that he enjoyed the construction, as well as keeping their machines going. "We actually did more carpentry than medicine for a while," Ted said, smiling. "We made most of the hospital furniture as well."

Then he related something that Denis would later conveniently recall. "Years ago, when Muriel and I were living on a shoestring, I bought an old car and managed to keep it running for seven years. I guess I like mechanical and electronic challenges."

That evening, when it came time for a bath, Ted's ingenuity impressed Denis again. The bathtub was an old dugout canoe with a plugged hole drilled in the bottom for release of the bath water. Olive whispered to Denis, "Now I can imagine what primitive missionary living must have been like for the Williamses!" Denis, himself, would subsequently appreciate Ted's versatility even more.

*****

It was also in 1950 that Hugh Trowell met Denis one day in the hospital library. Walking toward the back of the room together, Hugh asked, "Do you remember our visit on the train a few years ago when I said that some of my colleagues thought I was unduly obsessed with kwashiorkor and nutrition?"

Denis remembered well that first conversation. "Yes, of course, I was fascinated with the work you had done on this disease. Why do you ask?"

Sitting on the corner of a table and leaning toward his friend, Hugh said, "I'd been hoping for the appointment as Professor of Medicine at the medical school. As you know, I've been in charge of the medical and children's wards for years, as well as being the only Fellow of the Royal College of Physicians in East Africa." Hugh looked down at his feet and spoke in a low voice. "But, I understand that a number of colleagues have thought I was too one-sided in my nutritional research and therefore unsuitable for the appointment. They recommended another name to the committee in London."

"I heard about this appointment and couldn't believe that you had been bypassed because of your nutritional research!" Denis looked at him earnestly as he continued, "The university board should be pleased that you are engaged in original work." The two friends sat unspeaking for a few moments.

"It's an enormous disappointment, Denis, but the Lord will help me be kind and friendly with the man appointed to the position," Hugh said, picking up a book to leave.

This is a true measure of Hugh's dedicated Christian character, thought Denis as he pushed open the door and left the library.

*****

In March of 1952, their third daughter, Rachel, was born in the Mengo Hospital. Three months before, however, Olive had developed hepatitis with jaundice. Denis was doubly concerned about her when the obstetrics professor talked privately with him. The last time this lady physician had dealt with an expectant mother with hepatitis, she reported, the baby had been stillborn.

At birth, Rachel weighed just five pounds but thankfully was a healthy, normal newborn. Three days later, Olive and the baby were transferred to the nearby European Hospital in Kampala. Five-year-old Judy had been admitted there the previous day, suspected of having poliomyelitis, with fever and a stiff neck. A polio epidemic was sweeping through the city.

Her recent bout with hepatitis, in addition to worry over Judy, led Olive to suffer a postpartum depression. This was indeed a difficult time for Denis, since three-year-old Cassy was simultaneously sick at home with a stomach upset. He had to leave her in the care of Yusedi, their new, dependable Christian ayah. As Judy recovered from her illness with no complication, she was allowed to come into Olive's room. Toward the end of their three-week hospitalization, Cassy was also brought in from time to time to join them.

After returning home, Olive was still not well, and ten months later her illness necessitated a second hospitalization. Friends, with the help of Yusedi, took care of the three children during her absence. Denis was confident that Olive would recover completely with the change Laragh would afford, for they were soon due their second home leave.

And Laragh did work wonders for Olive with the love showered on her by Granny Burkitt. Once more the children enjoyed their Irish fairyland. Judy had forgotten "Alice" and "Echo House" of the previous visit. This time, the little girls took over an old shed on the grounds which they named "Forget-Me-Not Cottage." Here they played house and invited the grown-ups to tea, excitedly serving them "fairy sandwiches" and doll-sized cups of make-believe tea.

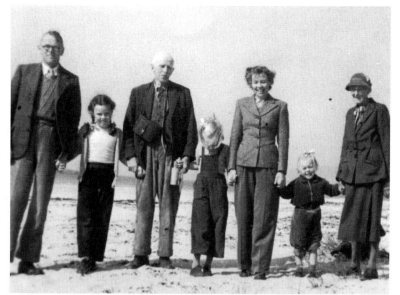

*Three generations of Burkitts enjoy an outing together at the seashore.
Left to right: Denis, Judy, Jim Burkitt, Cassy, Olive, Rachel and Gwen Burkitt.*

Granny's beautiful flower arrangements and Grandpa's constant variety of crisp, fresh vegetables from his kitchen garden were good therapy for the whole family, who once more relished the quiet beauty and warm homeyness of Laragh.

"Come, Olive, and bring Judy and Cassy too," Gwen Burkitt said one morning as she came back into the house with a bundle of dew-sparkling daffodils and snowdrops. "I'm going into Enniskillen to sell the flowers for a bit of pin-money."

Olive looked at Denis with surprise. It was news that her mother-in-law sold anything in the market. "I'd like to come along," Olive agreed.

"If you don't mind, dear, could you help me carry this basket with egg custard and a jug of soup for a sick cottage lady?" Granny packed the two articles in a shallow wicker basket and picked up the daffodils. "We'll stop there on our way to town."

"That's so thoughtful of you, mother dear," Olive said, admiring her sweet, gentle mother-in-law. "Come girls, let's go riding in the car with Granny." Olive opened the back door.

When she returned from town, Olive smiled as she privately told Denis of Granny's one desire. On the way to town, she had confided to Olive, "There's just one thing I'd like Jim to do for me. I'd like him to cut a door through the dining room into the kitchen garden attached to the house. Then I could go into the glass house easily and get winter vegetables without having to go outside in the weather."

"That sounds like a good idea. Why doesn't he do it?" Olive had asked.

"He says it costs too much." Gwen Burkitt wasn't complaining. She was just reporting facts.

*****

While on this leave, Denis took a few days to go over to England and visit his brother, Robin. As surgeons will, they began comparing typical cases in their surgical practices. They later continued their comparison of cases by mail, finding widely differing emergency abdominal surgeries encountered in England and Uganda. Denis never saw acute appendicitis, gall bladder disease, diverticular disease of the colon, or even hemorrhoids, all of which were common in Robin's practice. They decided to co-author a paper comparing the surgical diseases found in the two countries. Denis presented the information in a lecture at the inauguration of the East African Association of Surgeons in Nairobi. It was later published in a 1952 *East African Medical Journal,* his fifth published medical article since coming to Africa in 1946.

Little did the doctor-brothers imagine that they were touching on diseases of Western civilization rarely seen in the Third World, a subject which would become of major interest and an eventual research project for Denis. But before pursuing nutrition in global medicine, Denis was destined to engage in unusual cancer research which would bring both "Burkitt" and "Kampala" into worldwide prominence.

6

ENCOUNTER WITH A UNIQUE CANCER

Waiting to see Denis, who was just completing an ordinary morning patient visitation at the Mulago Hospital in 1957, Dr. Hugh Trowell asked if he would examine a problem case on the children's ward. The two doctors left the surgery ward and walked out into the bright African sunlight under a covered walkway connecting the low buildings. As they entered the pediatric unit, Hugh led Denis to the bedside of a five-year-old boy with deforming swellings on both sides of his upper and lower jaws.

One look at the pitifully disfigured face and Denis knew there was no hope for the child. However, he went through the motions of examining the opened mouth, palpating for lymph nodes in the neck, and scrutinizing the child's x-rays. Since the African child understood no English, Denis spoke openly to Trowell. "This is certainly a puzzling picture," he said, examining the boy's opened mouth. "It has to be a cancer. Look at the way all the teeth in both jaws are displaced. They seem to be attached only to the gums."

"Have you ever seen a tumor in all four quadrants of the jaws?" Trowell asked.

"Never, Hugh!" Denis was emphatic, and turning to Trowell, admitted, "I can't really make sense out of what I'm seeing. How can a tumor spread from one side of the jaw to the other, or more importantly, from the upper to the lower jaw? It's certainly hard to explain." Burkitt rested his hand on the boy's shoulder. "The fact that there are no enlarged lymph nodes in the neck only adds to the enigma. There's nothing I can do for the boy except take a biopsy, or has one already been done?" he asked, noting a small, partially-healed scar under the boy's left jaw.

72

"A biopsy was taken," Hugh informed him, making a note in the chart, "and the report is a 'small round-cell sarcoma.' Actually, that doesn't tell us very much, except that it's a highly malignant form of cancer."

They walked away from the bedside. "Thanks for showing me the case, Hugh, but I haven't a clue," Denis apologized.

"I didn't really expect you to come up with a startling suggestion for treatment," Hugh replied, "but I thought you might like to see this baffling case."

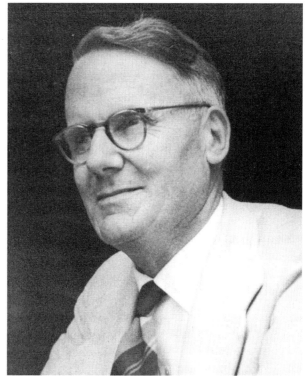

Good friend, Doctor Hugh Trowell

"This is the gloomy part of medicine," Denis said as he left the ward with Trowell, "especially when it involves children."

*****

One of Burkitt's responsibilities as consulting surgeon at Mulago was to make routine surgical rounds in outlying district hospitals. Several weeks later, he went to the Jinja Hospital near the source of the Nile, about fifty miles east of Kampala. He and Olive had attended a ceremony at Jinja a few years earlier, when Princess Elizabeth, later Queen Elizabeth II, opened the great hydroelectric system which would supply electricity to the whole of Uganda and much of Kenya.

In the midst of making surgical rounds at Jinja one morning, Denis's attention was suddenly riveted on a child he noticed through the open window of the ward. There on the lawn outside, sitting on his mother's lap, was another child with a grotesquely swollen face. Denis immediately excused himself and strode outdoors to examine the child. How could it be? Here was a second child with exactly the same features as Hugh Trowell's patient, with deforming tumors in all four quadrants of the jaws. In fact, the swellings prevented this boy from closing his mouth completely.

Denis persuaded the mother to bring the child and ride back to Kampala with him for a more complete examination. As he drove back through the dark forests interspersed with extensive sugar cane fields, his mind raced. *Hugh told me that the biopsy on his case showed a "small round-cell sarcoma."* (This is a term used by pathologists to describe a highly malignant cancer composed of a single-cell type with uniform-sized nuclei and scant cytoplasm). *As I have time, I think I'll pull the hospital charts on all cases of jaw tumors in children.*

After admitting the boy to the children's ward at Mulago Hospital, Denis examined him more thoroughly and was surprised to find that he also had lumps in his abdomen. *These are doubtless also tumors—but with jaw cancer spreading to the abdomen? That's a bit unusual. In fact, while I'm looking up cases, I'll examine the records of all tumors of children, regardless of type, and see if there are ones similar to these two cases.* He was now more eager than ever to start reviewing hospital records of children with this unusual condition.

Sure enough, as he examined old records, he did indeed find other cases of children with the strange jaw tumors. All these stricken children had eventually died, and postmortem examination had been done on a number of them. Microscopic examination invariably showed the same picture, all "small round-cell sarcomas."

Many of the children with jaw tumors also had abdominal tumors. But even more intriguing were cases that appeared to be of the same type of cancer but involving many organs—thyroid gland, adrenal glands, kidneys, eyes, testes of boys, ovaries of girls, as well as breast tissue, long bones, even the pericardium (the fibrous sac enclosing the heart). He noted that some of the cases with widespread tumors did not involve the jaws at all. Strange to say, the tumor usually spared peripheral lymph nodes, although occasionally it involved abdominal lymph nodes.

The diagnoses of the tumor varied. If it involved the eye, it had been called a "retinoblastoma;" if the adrenal, a "neuroblastoma;" if the ovary, a "granulosa-cell tumor;" in long bones, "Ewing's tumor;" and in the kidney, "Wilms' tumor." Some of the children had died with total paralysis and loss of sensation in the legs, evidently due to pressure from the tumors interfering with the blood supply to the spinal cord.

Actually, all of these tumors had the same appearance under the microscope, being composed of "small round cells." *But*, reasoned Denis, *why should several of these different tumors sometimes occur together in various combinations in a single child? There's no reason for a "neuroblastoma," a "retinoblastoma," a "Wilms' tumor" to all occur in the same child! Interestingly, the jaw tumors are not always associated with multiple tumors in other sites.* The more he thought about it, the more he concluded, *If several of the lesions occur together, one should suspect a common cause. Could all of these tumors be part of the same picture and have the same ultimate cause?*

"Wilms'," "retinoblastoma," "neuroblastoma" were all standard separate diagnoses in pathology books. However, these texts had never described the combined picture of the cancer Denis was now researching.

He made a note in his diary, which he had recently begun to keep again. "June 1, 1957: I presented the jaw tumors as well as congenital limb deformities in children at today's morning staff meeting." He had been working on congenital defects at the time and was considering the two medical problems of about equal importance. This was his first recorded note concerning the enigmatic tumor.

Several months later, on October 8, he wrote, "Encouraging session with John (Croot) and Ian (McAdam) over the jaw syndrome." Soon everyone in the hospital knew that Burkitt was studying the jaw tumors, and his interest in the subject was relayed by word-of-mouth. Before long, hospitals and clinics throughout Uganda were sending him children with jaw tumors.

A few doctors on the hospital staff told him outright he was talking "baloney" in trying to make something special of the cases. Denis challenged a pathologist friend to examine slides of the tumor removed from the kidney, ovary and eye, and identify the tumor as being a specific cancer of the organ involved.

"Can you tell me from the appearance of the tumor under the microscope from what organ these were removed?" Denis asked. The pathologist was stumped. He couldn't differentiate the cancers as specific to certain organs.

None of these unusual cases escaped Denis's camera. At frequent intervals he took a roll or two of film to the hospital x-ray darkroom to develop and print his black and white pictures. He always accomplished the final washing process in the bathtub at home. Not infrequently Olive would remind him, "It's bath-time for the girls, Denis. Haven't these prints washed long enough?"

Little Cassy, peering into the tub, might exclaim, "What's wrong with that boy's face, Mummy? Look at that poor little girl's crooked leg. Why does Daddy take all these funny pictures?"

Denis would quickly gather the array of bizarre medical prints and spread them out to dry, saying, "Daddy's doing some special studies to try to help these poor children, Cassy."

On October 11, Denis wrote in his diary, "Difficult obstructive session with a colleague over jaw tumor." In fact, the colleague got up and left the meeting in anger, but Denis was undaunted. He drew an age graph distribution of the tumors. It was strange indeed. The tumor never appeared to occur before the age of two. The peak occurrence was at eight years, and the disease almost disappeared by the age of twelve. Regardless of whether the tumor was in the jaw, kidney, eye, bone, or a combination of these or other sites, the age graph was the same. This fact again suggested to him a common cause of all the tumors.

He tried to make sense of the findings. *Neuroblastoma of the adrenal gland sometimes spreads to the skull. Could it be that this is a neuroblastoma spreading to the jaws instead of to the cranium?* He had already decided that the tumor didn't necessarily originate in the jaws, because it didn't always involve the jaws. Neither did the cancer always involve the adrenal glands. Nothing seemed to fit right in this medical jigsaw puzzle!

*****

As Denis and Olive sat on their veranda one late afternoon, admiring the garden stretching down the hill, he complimented her, saying, "You've really done wonderfully well in providing beautiful flowers for the house, just as Mummy always did at Laragh." For Olive, working in the flower beds was a joy, just as it had always been for Gwen Burkitt. She had found a variety of familiar flowers which did well in spite of the tropical weather.

Olive looked over her garden with some satisfaction, her eyes coming to rest on the children's playhouse. Turning to Denis, she commented, "How the children have enjoyed the Wendy house you built out of packing crates, Denis! The wood has weathered nicely, so it looks well in the garden setting."

Smiling, he recalled, "It was fun building it in sections. The girls had no idea what I was making and storing in the garage until Christmas morning, when I took

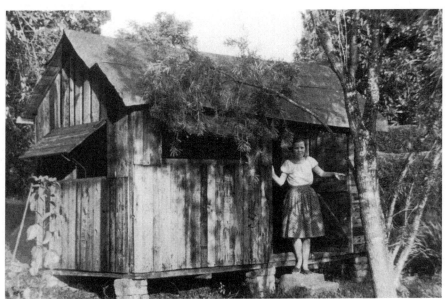

Judy stands at the door of the packing crate Wendy house.

it all out and began bolting the sections together." Ever since his schoolboy days, he had enjoyed carpentry.

Changing the subject, Olive reached for a book on the stand near her chair. "Denis, I've been reading your Uncle Roland's biography, *Under the Sun*, that we recently received. You remember that his associate, Dr. J. R. Gregory, told you he was going to write one." She was finding Uncle Roland such an interesting person, she wanted Denis to enjoy the book also and decided to pique his curiosity with a few choice portions. Turning the pages of the small book, she said, "I know you haven't had time to look at the book yet, but did you ever wonder what Uncle Roland's wife was like?"

"I didn't know very much about her," Denis admitted, "but I do know that she died of a brain tumor at rather a young age."

Olive filled in the background of how Roland Burkitt, upon completing his surgical training, had gone out to Nairobi on a trip and decided to set up his practice there. "Let me read some of it to you," she offered.

> After a short visit to England to purchase equipment, he returned and cast in his lot with the other pioneers. On the return voyage he met his future wife. She was a tall, slim, graceful woman, with even attractive features, and a charming expression eloquent of her character, who would attract attention in any company. She was traveling as companion to Lady Inverclyde who was going to join her husband, the Governor of Gibraltar.

> Miss Anita Carter, as she was then, had many suitors on board and was much sought after as a companion and dancing partner. Burkitt was at a great disadvantage as he had never danced in his life, nor could his looks be highly commended, but he pursued the woman of his choice with great persistence all day and paid her every possible attention. When the tender came alongside to convey Lady Inverclyde and her companion ashore Burkitt was all ready to accompany them, but this was forbidden. In the few minutes at his disposal on the gangway he succeeded in extracting a promise of marriage from the blushing maiden, and when the ship sailed on he astonished many of the better favored and, as they thought, more desirable young men by announcing his engagement.

> She joined him within the year and shared his life in Kenya, taking the rough with the smooth, mostly happy but often resenting his eccentricities which she found irksome. She tried hard to protect

him against overwork and made no secret of her displeasure when he was pestered with calls after a hard day, especially if they came in the late evening or night. Her anger was turned against him, when he insisted on taking the call.

Denis interrupted, saying, "After his wife died, he stayed on in Nairobi, and never remarried."

"I would say that his poor wife put up with a lot. Listen to this," Olive continued to read.

> In the days of Mrs. Burkitt very often he got home to find a tea-party in full swing arranged by his wife, who never dared to ask his permission as he invariably said "No." Mrs. Burkitt, who had spent a comparatively dull day doing the chores of a Kenya housewife, could not be expected to live the life of a recluse and, in addition, she had to return hospitality. When it was inevitable and the guests were assembled, Burkitt would enter into the party spirit and spare no pains to entertain the guests. As soon as he could get away, he would proceed on his rounds, accompanied by his wife and his son.

"You mean he took his wife and son every evening on rounds?" Denis laughed in disbelief. "Aren't you glad I don't take you and the girls with me on medical rounds?"

Olive smiled and then skipped to another anecdote about Roland and Anita Burkitt which she thought especially humorous.

> Mrs. Burkitt was a particularly beautiful woman, tall, slender, graceful and well featured. In spite of these assets she found it difficult to satisfy all her husband's whims. What beautiful woman does not wish to create a sensation in the fashion of her day? It was not possible for Mrs. Burkitt to do this while skirts were worn short, as her husband would not countenance her following such a fashion. It takes a very clever man to outdo a determined woman, and Mrs. Burkitt met what she considered to be an impossible situation by having her dresses fitted with two belts, one of which enabled her to wear them long to please her husband, and one which held them up to the fashionable length to please the dictates of fashion. It caused immense amusement to her friends to see her skirt being lengthened by a chuck the moment Dr. Burkitt appeared on the scene.

"Well, it looks as though I must learn how the Burkitts are supposed to conduct themselves," Denis said, with a twinkle in his eye.

Flipping pages, Olive came to another page with the corner turned down. "You've got to read this, Denis, you'll really enjoy knowing more about your uncle."

> He was an early riser, and every morning he was up at or before dawn reading in his study wrapped in a warm Jaegar dressing-gown over his pajamas. In cold weather he put on socks and sometimes a muffler. For two hours he divided his time into Bible study and reading scientific medical journals or books. If an urgent call came during those hours or in the night he would set off to see the patient in this unconventional garb, surmounted by a sun-helmet.

> At 6 o'clock his African servant brought him a large pot of tea and he drank several cups well sweetened. The tea was intended to wake him up, and the sugar to give him energy. If he had guests staying in the house it gave him great pleasure, if they would join him at this hour and listen to his discourse on some abstruse theological problem. The study of the Scriptures and the origin and history of words used in the Bible was a constant source of interest to him. To take but one example, the substitution of the word "even" for "and" in the Grace gives a new and more emphatic meaning to those beautiful words: "The Grace of our Lord, Jesus Christ, even the Love of God, even the Fellowship of the Holy Ghost, be with us all." He would point out how each idea meant the same thing and was merely tautological in order to be emphatic. It is noteworthy how often the word "and" in the Bible is better translated as "even."

"Well, listen to that!" Denis suddenly leaned forward in his chair. "When I was a teenager, Uncle Roland came for a visit. He asked Robin and me how many meanings of the word 'and' there were in Leviticus. To this very day, I thought he just had an odd twist of humor—but he really meant it! There evidently is at least one other meaning to the word!"

*****

In February 1958, Denis presented his first paper on jaw tumors at the annual meeting of the East African Surgeons in Kampala and stirred up some enthusiasm for the subject. He next worked up the material to submit for publication in the *British Journal of Surgery* in 1958 under the title, "Tumours Involving the Jaws in African Children." This aroused no general interest whatsoever in either the British or American readership. At the end of June, the director of the Cancer Research Unit from South Africa, Dr. George Oettle, visited Kampala, giving Denis the opportunity to talk with a cancer expert. He led Dr. Oettle to the pediatric ward and showed him a child with four-quadrant jaw tumors who also had lumps in the abdomen that could be easily felt. They reviewed the x-rays together. Then Denis took him to his office and showed him photographs of many similar cases with massively swollen jaws.

"These are all 'small round-cell sarcomas.' What do you think?" Denis asked.

"I can tell you at least one thing for sure," said Oettle, putting the photographs back on the desk. "This tumor doesn't exist in South Africa."

Upon hearing such a definite statement from Oettle, who should know, Denis mulled this idea in his head for several days. *Could there be a **geographical distribution** of this strange cancer? Parasitic diseases, of course, often have geographic distribution—yes, and primary cancer of the liver is more prevalent in certain areas of Africa and Asia than in other areas of the world. If it's true that this tumor doesn't occur in South Africa, there must be a good reason. Some studies on the geographic incidence of these jaw tumors are certainly indicated.* Upon reviewing the jaw tumor records again, he found most of their tumors at Mulago were coming from north and east Uganda, with relatively fewer cases from the south and west.

At the next weekly staff meeting, Denis eagerly shared his newest findings with his colleagues. Lifting a board with a map attached, Denis began by saying, "I've prepared this preliminary map of Uganda and designated

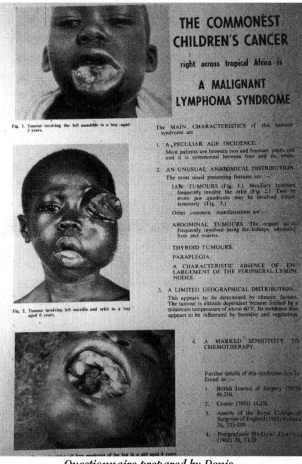

Questionnaire prepared by Denis.

with pins the home area of each patient suffering from the tumor. As you can see, the cases appear to be coming mainly from the north and east parts of Uganda. When Dr. Oettle was here recently, he told me quite definitely that there were none of these cases in South Africa. I'm beginning to think the tumor might have a geographic distribution."

"Very interesting, Denis. What do you propose to do next?" Ian McAdam was always supportive of his work.

"I'm thinking it might be worthwhile," Denis suggested, "to make up some illustrated leaflets describing the tumor and send these widely throughout Africa."

"Sounds like a good idea," fellow surgeon, John Croot agreed. "How will you distribute the questionnaires?"

"We have lists of government and mission hospitals," Denis said, pleased with the favorable response, "but I suppose the biggest problem now is financing the project."

With this last remark, a colleague who had been opposing Denis got up from his chair rather noisily and walked out of the conference.

Wishing to relieve the tension, Ian assured Denis, "I'm sure we can get a government grant for the printing and postage of your leaflet. I'll see what can be done. Why don't you prepare the questionnaire, including a picture of one or two of these children?"

Needing no further encouragement, Denis selected three photographs: one of a child with a four-jaw tumor showing displaced teeth; another with a massively swollen left jaw; and one with both a jaw and an eye tumor. He included brief descriptions of possible organ involvement, as well as a questionnaire which asked: "Do you see this jaw tumor? Do you see the tumor in other sites?"

Before long, two government grants came in for £15 and £10 (total $75.00). This was sufficient for frugal Denis to get 1,000 leaflets printed as well as to pay for postage. He mailed these all over Africa, handed them out at conferences, and gave them to all medical visitors. In anticipation of receiving answers to his survey, he fastened a large map of Africa to the wall of his office.

*****

As Denis opened the back door of their house one morning, he called the girls to hurry and get into the car so that he could drive them to school. After he backed out of the garage, the three girls jumped into the front seat with him and reminded him to pick up some other children. After three additional children climbed into the back seat, Denis drove, lost in thought, down the Kampala street and turned right at the end of the avenue. Suddenly, the unusually quiet six children burst into laughter.

"It worked!" screamed Cassy, "Daddy, you forgot we were even in the car and turned up to the European Hospital instead of the school!"

"You little rascals!" chuckled Denis, as he stopped and turned the car around. He knew they had purposely tricked him by being so quiet he forgot they were with him. Now, every spare moment, his thoughts were focused on the intriguing jaw-tumor riddle.

On July 3 Denis noted in his diary, "Very excited over findings at a postmortem of jaw tumor case. Other cancer deposits in the body confirm my idea that all of it is the same tumor. My colleague who always differs with me felt these were unrelated tumors occurring in different sites."

In the midst of all this medical excitement, a letter from Denis's mother on August 27 caused considerable anxiety in the family.

> Dear Daddy is almost bedridden and having considerable pain, but
> still mentally clear. He is so ready to go. I wonder if he will be able
> to write you again. I thank God for him.

James Burkitt had just passed his 88th birthday. Their next home leave was still eight months away. Another family situation in the fall involved twelve-year-old Judy, who must leave home for a school in Kenya. This parting was especially traumatic for Olive.

Early in January a letter from Gwen Burkitt indicated that Denis's father was sinking rapidly. Now it was only four months until their home leave, and once again they wondered if he would still be at Laragh when they returned.

Complications in Denis's professional life also surfaced. On January 31, 1959, Denis entered another reference to the jaw tumors in his diary: "My colleague who has always disputed my findings today spoke at the International Cancer Conference on the subject of *Jaw Tumors* without any reference to my prior work. I must seek grace not to feel touchy."

Early in February, Denis had a long discussion with Dr. Greg O'Conor, a new pathologist at Makerere. This brilliant young man had come out to work in a Catholic Hospital before transferring to Kampala. One would never imagine this unassuming young man had come from a wealthy family, their means derived from his father's invention of Formica. Greg, after carefully examining the enigmatic tumor from many sites in the body, concurred with Denis that the various cancer deposits all represented the same tumor spreading widely throughout the body. The other pathologists also agreed with him now.

Meanwhile, many replies to Denis's jaw tumor leaflet poured into his office. With each response, he inserted a new pin with a colored paper flag into the large map of Africa. Daughters Cassy and Rachel often helped their daddy stick pins in the areas where the cancer was observed. As the months passed, a distinct "belt" across tropical Africa began to appear on the map, approximately ten degrees above and ten degrees below the equator. Strangely, a "tail" extended from the belt and ran down the African east coast. The mystery of the strange cancer was growing ever more fascinating.

The following month, on March 31, a wire received from Robin stated:

DADDY PASSED PEACEFULLY THIS MORNING (MARCH 30).

How sad this message was for the family that was to start on their 1959 home leave the next morning. There would be no Grandpa to meet them at the Enniskillen station, and Laragh would never be the same without the quiet, gentle man who characteristically wore his binoculars like a badge about his neck.

*****

At home in Laragh, early in June, Denis received a surprising letter from his dissenting colleague saying he also now accepted the fact that the multiple tumors in various sites, including the jaw, were all the same cancer.

In mid-June, Denis, accompanied by nine-year-old Cassy, who enjoyed bicycling in the country with her father, rode out over the rolling Irish hills. But this time the brakes on Jim Burkitt's forty-year-old bicycle, retrieved from the barn, failed as Denis was going downhill. When he tried to slow the bicycle with his foot on the front tire, his shoe caught in the wheel spokes, throwing him over the handlebars and knocking him unconscious. Cassy, fearing her father was dead, raced on her bike the short way to a friend's house to phone her mother.

When Olive arrived in the car a few minutes later, Denis had regained consciousness but found he couldn't move his right elbow, which was badly smashed. Since the only surgeon in Enniskillen was unavailable, he simply had the entire arm secured in a cast by the resident physician. His immediate fear was that a stiff arm might interfere with his surgery or photography. Knowing his elbow injury required expert orthopedic attention, he had Olive drive him to Belfast the next day. There he found an orthopedist who agreed to manipulate the joint fracture under anesthesia rather than employ the newer method of using screws and plates.

Denis cared little for the satisfaction of a cosmetically perfect result. He desired only good function. Realizing the seriousness of the injury and its future effect on his entire professional life, he prayed, *Nevertheless, not my will, but Thine be done.* After returning home, he faithfully raised the arm several times a day by a pulley apparatus he'd rigged over the limb of a beech tree in the garden. Fortunately, the fracture healed with good function, rewarding his early exercise to prevent stiffness.

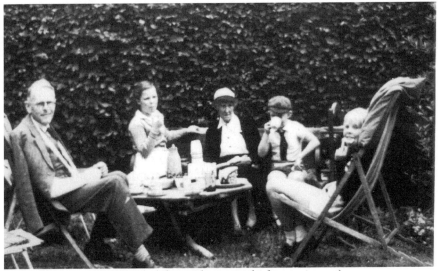

At Laragh, left to right: Denis (right arm in cast),
Judy, Granny Burkitt, Rachel and Cassy.

The injury didn't prevent him in August from enjoying with the girls a before-breakfast climb to the top of a nearby mountain. They returned, exhilarated and happy, to a picnic breakfast which Olive had cooked over a fire at the foot of the mountain. What a wonderful, carefree time for them all. Denis noted with satisfaction that his mother savored every moment of their visit, although they both dreaded the upcoming parting. Within a couple of weeks, it would be time to return to Uganda.

Leaving Granny at Laragh was difficult for the whole family, for after the death of Grandpa, she was physically more fragile and had little desire to live. They felt this might be the last time they would see her. Her faithful maid of many years, Lizzie, would still be her companion, so she would not be alone. They all cried as the car pulled out of the driveway, leaving behind the slight, white-haired little figure on the front steps.

Denis's heart was really torn, for in spite of the sad parting with his mother, he did look forward with anticipation to getting back to Uganda. In London, he met and had lunch with Jack Darling, who was also on furlough and had just learned of his appointment to the surgery department at Mulago. Denis, pleased that they'd soon be working together, filled him in a bit on his jaw-cancer project.

"This is a tumor which puzzles everyone," Denis told him. "I brought some microscopic slides of the tumor back to England with me. I've been carrying them around to the London teaching hospitals and have shown them to a dozen different pathologists. I've received about eleven different diagnoses!"

Jack sensed his friend's frustration, saying he had no doubt that one day he'd solve the problem. He added, "Knowing you, Denis, the tumor's mystery only makes the research all the more intriguing."

Denis looked at his friend, but his thoughts were elsewhere. Already he was formulating new ideas for tracking the unusual cancer.

7

NAILING DOWN A "LYMPHOMA"

Another development awaited Denis on his return to Mulago in September 1959. The new pathologist, Dr. Greg O'Conor, while intensely studying the jaw tumors, had classified them as a **"lymphoma,"** [a lymphoma cancer is composed of primitive lymphocytes, a type of white blood cell]. Greg had reviewed all the childhood cancers in the Kampala Cancer Registry and found fifty percent of all African childhood cancers were these lymphomas! This was an extremely high incidence of lymphoma compared with six to eight percent of all types of lymphomas in American childhood cancer.

Denis was soon busying himself getting his map of Africa up to date and adding many more cases from replies to his questionnaires which had come in during his absence. The tumor pattern was even more definite now, with a distinct equatorial belt and secondary tail running down the east coast. He somehow managed to squeeze his exciting tumor research into a full surgery schedule. How thankful he was that his elbow injury had not impaired his surgical skills.

He soon learned that his friend, Jack Darling, was preceding his wife Beryl and their children to Kampala. Upon Jack's arrival, Denis and Olive opened their home to him rather than let him live in a hostel. When Jack began unpacking and arranging furniture in their assigned house, Olive volunteered her help to make it a comfortable home for his family.

Then, in a diary entry of October 26, Denis expressed a new concern: "Very worried after reading an article authored by my colleague who has previously opposed my work. He is publishing much of my work without any acknowledgment to me. Nearly spoiled my day. This shows a sensitive and very much alive 'self' which should be crucified." The next day, Denis confided in his diary: "Far too concerned over my colleague's publishing results of my research. Jesus made Himself of 'no reputation.' Yet I'm afraid of losing some kudos. He said, 'If a man takes your coat, give your cloak also.' After all, as the apostle Paul wrote, 'What have I that I did not receive?' " On October 28, he added this succinct note: "Feeling better over my colleague."

Meanwhile he was co-authoring a paper, more complete than the one previously published in the *British Journal of Surgery*, entitled, "Malignant Lymphoma in African Children." Denis described the clinical features of the disease, providing a map of the "lymphoma belt" as well as the then-known distribution of the tumor in East Africa. Greg O'Conor, in a second part, covered pathological features and microscopic descriptions of the tumor. The two men completed the article and mailed it for publication in May 1960.

During that same month, his friend Hugh Trowell told him, "Denis, I've decided to retire. I've been in Africa a little over thirty years now."

"You're too young to retire, Hugh," Denis objected.

"Oh, I'm only retiring from medicine!" he assured him. "I've had a lifelong desire to become an ordained minister of the Gospel. So, I'm returning to England to study for the ministry." Dr. Trowell thought he was leaving his medical prac-

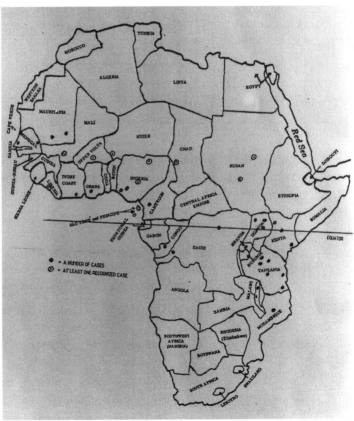

Map of Africa showing the lymphoma belt.

87

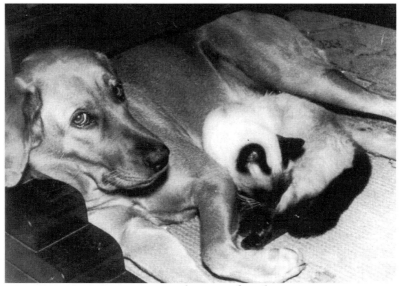

Ranee and Siamese friend.

tice behind him; however, some years later, Burkitt would again play a part in Trowell's life, when they would become heavily involved together in medical research.

With the Trowells leaving Mulago Hill, Cassy Burkitt had one big concern. "When the Trowells go, what will happen to the crested cranes in their garden?" Cassy was the "pet girl," loving every creature.

"Why don't you ask them about the birds, dear?" Olive suggested. "But please don't offer to take them, for we have enough pets of our own!"

At different times the children had rabbits, a tortoise, a chameleon, and a pet turkey. Cassy, especially, adored them all and was diligent in caring for them. Lately she had been reading up on dogs and had begun begging for a golden Labrador retriever. Denis and Olive, agreeing that the girls really should have a dog, had ordered a puppy from a kennel in Kenya. Ecstatic, Cassy read up on how to make a dog house and had one ready when the puppy arrived. But to her disappointment, the puppy had already far outgrown its newly-fabricated quarters. Never mind! The more important task now was to find a suitable name for the dog. The girls decided that "Ranee," an Indian designation for a queen, was a fitting name for their newest pet, which soon became fast friends with their Siamese cat.

One day, Denis arrived home from work to hear quite a story from Olive. While the girls were in school, Olive had heard noisy squeaking from the white-mice cage, fixed to a post of the veranda. On investigating, she had found a snake inside the cage. It had already devoured several mice and had retreated into the mice's sleeping quarters for a nap. Two squeaking survivors trembled at the far end of the cage.

Olive, in a quandary as to what to do, finally plugged any possible escape routes the snake might find and waited until Denis returned from work. His solution was to drop a chloroform-drenched ball of cotton over the snake, which consequently failed to awaken from its nap.

"No more mice, girls," Olive said, to which they heartily agreed.

"I take care of many more patients for the treatment given for snake bites than for snake bites," Denis advised them, trying to calm the fears of his whole female family, who were afraid of snakes. "Many times a tourniquet is applied after a snake bite and never loosened. I've had to amputate a few gangrenous extremities as a result."

*****

On August 24, 1960 Denis recorded sad words in his diary: "News of dear Mummy's passing last night. We wouldn't have it otherwise. Thank the Lord for all dear Mummy has been to us." On August 30 he wrote further: "Poignant letter from Robin. All about dear Mummy's passing. Died in peace. Need guidance of what to do with Laragh."

Denis thought with gratitude of the devotion and care to his aging parents given for years by two friends. His mother had, many years before, taken into their home a teenaged orphan boy, Dick Smith, who had slept on a couch in his father's office. When the senior Burkitts needed help in later years, Dick did everything he could for them, even taking care of their car and garden after his working hours. At the same time their maid of many years, Lizzie, faithfully stayed with them until they both passed away. Denis rested in the thought that these faithful friends had lovingly cared for his dear parents. There was nothing he could do now but once more totally submerge himself in his cancer project.

*****

The apparent geographical distribution of the lymphoma was, of itself, a unique finding. What did it mean? As he and Greg suggested in their recently submitted article, they must consider the possibility of a viral agent causing the cancer. But up to this time, no virus had ever been found as a cause of human cancer. Denis felt it was only a matter of time until someone would make such a discovery, since viruses had for many years been identified as causing several animal cancers. The possible virus etiology of human cancer was currently a "hot subject," with many investigators working on it.

Denis regarded his first challenge to be a determination of the factor or factors causing the strange geographical distribution of this African tumor. What were the local conditions in areas where the tumor was prevalent, and how might these factors contribute to a cancer? There were yet many missing features of his medical enigma. Even though he'd had a good response to his questionnaires, he was not entirely satisfied, for there were geographical gaps in the information they provided. He was now sure that only an extensive fact-finding trip could supply the needed answers, and this would require considerable planning and fund-raising.

Frequently on Sunday afternoons when they had a few hours for relaxation, Denis and Jack Darling took long walks together, accompanied by Ranee, the retriever. As they hiked up and down the many hills surrounding Kampala, discussing the lymphoma project, Denis privately aired his concern that some of their medical colleagues opposed his research. In spite of trying to ignore these criticisms, the very fact that there was not complete openness and harmony, disturbed him. Deep in his heart, he knew that he should not let it bother him. He rarely discussed the situation, even with Olive.

✳✳✳✳✳

At the end of October, 1960 Dr. Joseph Burchenal from the Sloane-Kettering Institute in New York visited Kampala. Since Burchenal's specialty was cancer chemotherapy, he had come to see if any of the cancer chemotherapeutic agents could be successfully used in the newly described childhood lymphoma. After examining several of the afflicted children, he sat with Burkitt late one afternoon, discussing what plan to use.

"As you may know, in New York, we've been having fairly good success in treating leukemia with chemotherapy, specifically using Methotrexate," Burchenal began.

"But none of our lymphoma cases have ever developed leukemia," Denis commented with some skepticism.

"Even so, because lymphoma and lymphocytic leukemia are closely related," Burchenal urged, "I think we might find regression of these tumors, using this drug. It's certainly worth a try."

"I agree. These poor children don't stand a chance with any other type of therapy," Denis said. "What program do you recommend?"

Burchenal shifted on his seat and flipped through the papers of a protocol in his hand. "Our experience has been to treat the children to maximum tolerance. They get pretty sick, but it's the only way to destroy the cancer. We treat with several courses."

Denis placed the tips of his spread fingers together, pursed his lips, and thought for a minute. "I have two children in the hospital right now that we can begin therapy on. They've both been biopsied, and they're proven cases of the lymphoma."

The next day, Denis, under the direction of Burchenal, began treating a little boy named "Israel." They could hardly believe how dramatically the tumor regressed after a single injection of Methotrexate. The child often came to the Burkitt home, and the whole family followed his progress. However, the tumor gradually began to enlarge again, and before long the child died. This moved not only Denis nearly to tears, but the whole family as well. With trepidation, he gave a second little boy the drug. Again, almost miraculously, the tumor melted away. This time the cancer did not recur after many weeks. Denis was jubilant.

He acquired and began using, on a trial basis, a second drug, Endoxan (cyclophosphamide), also with good results. Before long he admitted to the hospital a little girl with a small jaw lesion. He gave her the first course of Endoxan, but in the middle of the night the child's mother came to the pediatric ward and carried

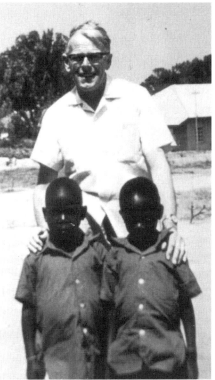

Denis with two patients "cured" by chemotherapy.

her away. *What a shame!* thought Denis, *she could have been cured if she'd only had a complete course of the drug.* Some time later, the child returned. Surprisingly, she had no evidence of the cancer and remained well, apparently cured.

Fortuitously, Denis had found that cures were possible with minimal drug therapy, a revolutionary idea. *Evidently*, he reasoned, *if a relatively small amount of chemical eradicates the bulk of the tumor, the body's own immune system can then take over to eliminate the remaining cancer cells.*

Greatly encouraged by these initial, apparent cures, Denis wrote to several pharmaceutical companies, requesting free medicines for experimental purposes. His approach was that since no hospital in tropical Africa had x-radiation therapy available, the chemical alone would be used in treatment of the lymphoma, thus proving the true efficacy of the medicine. Lederle Laboratories immediately sent $300.00 worth of drugs as a starter. The chemotherapeutic approach to the disease had been successfully launched.

During 1960, Dr. Dennis Wright joined the Makerere Medical School faculty. He was an English pathologist and a specialist in "histochemistry," the study of tissue

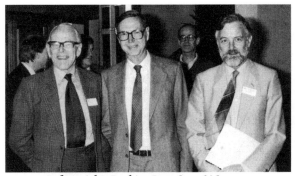

Left to right: Burkitt, Drs. Greg O'Connor and Dennis Wright. Picture taken years later.

and cell chemistry. Dr. Wright heard about the strange childhood cancer soon after arriving in Kampala, and initially had little interest in it. But before long, it became his duty to perform several postmortem examinations of children dying of the tumor.

To better study the cancer cells, Dr. Wright made fresh tissue imprints by gently touching the cut surface of a tumor to clean glass slides and then staining the tumor imprints with standard dyes. Examining these stained imprints, he was surprised to find the cancer cells were all of one type, with a characteristic appearance different from any human lymphoma he had previously seen. The cytoplasm of the lymphoid cells stained a very dark blue color and contained small fat droplets (vacuoles). **Wright proved by his close microscopic study of the tumor cells that this African cancer was a new, unknown type of lymphoma.**

✱✱✱✱✱

Months later, one evening near Christmas, Olive and the girls finished decorating a tree and arranging presents beneath it. Before sending the children to bed, she told them the Christmas story of the birth of Jesus and how astonished shepherds had visited the newborn Savior. As she and the girls sat in their living room, they noticed a light approaching and heard voices. Olive opened the French doors. Outside was a group of Africans. One held a lighted lantern on a pole, another held a sheep by a rope around its neck. An elderly woman stood in front of the group.

"I've brought a Christmas present for the doctor," the woman explained. "The doctor operated on me twice, and saved my life both times."

"Come in," Olive invited. "I was just telling the story of the first Christmas, when Jesus was born, and how the shepherds came with their sheep. Now you have brought us a sheep. The children will never forget this night or your present to the doctor," Olive exclaimed as she accepted the gift for her husband, for he, unfortunately, had been detained late at the hospital.

After they'd gone, Cassy, with wide-eyed wonder, said, "This is a special sheep. We mustn't kill the sheep and eat it. It's a Christmas sheep."

For several days, the little sheep was tethered in the garden, but finally Denis gave it to the hospital chaplain, Pastor Galiwango.

*****

By January 1961, news of the unusual childhood cancer had reached Sir Harold Himsworth, director of the British Medical Research Council in London. He came out to Kampala to see firsthand what its potentials were for research. As a result of an interview with Denis, he offered £150 ($450.00) toward the investigation. This was the first recognition of his studies by a scientific organization. Elated, Denis wrote in his diary on January 7: "The sun has shone on my work, but this creates dangers. Success is empty. I would rather be nearer the Lord. How to abound may be harder than how to be abased."

Himsworth immediately observed some confusion at the hospital as to who was actually the chief investigator of the lymphoma project, but Ian McAdam, successfully defended Denis as the original investigator. Ian recommended that Burkitt be appointed to direct all field studies on the tumor. Further, he requested a grant of £3,000 ($9,000.00) for three years. Denis marveled at how things were providentially working out for him.

A February 10 diary entry would one day become significant: "Met three U.S. doctors— one, C. Everett Koop— who seemed quite interested in the lymphomas." Denis would learn only later that the virus potential of the cancer had greatly impressed Dr. Koop, who was destined to become a future United States Surgeon General. When Koop returned to Philadelphia, he suggested to Werner and Gertrude Henle, a well-known virologist team working at his hospital, that the African lymphoma would be a good place to look for a human cancer virus.

Before his next home leave, now at eighteen-month intervals instead of three years, Denis planned his fact-finding safari through a part of Africa. What environmental factors on one side of the lymphoma belt boundary were different from those on the other side? Denis called this approach a "geographical biopsy" because he planned to note environmental factors on either side of the boundary.

He decided that the northern boundary was unsatisfactory, for its population dwindled and finally disappeared in the desert. The southern boundary of West Africa was inappropriate as it ended in the Gulf of Guinea. A revolution in Angola made part of the southern boundary unsafe for travel. He narrowed his proposed route to the only reasonable and accessible region, the southeastern part of the lymphoma belt, the so-called "tail" on his map. Populations there were reasonably dense, roads were passable, and the countries were politically stable.

In this designated area, he intended to visit all medical facilities, both government and mission-operated, questioning doctors and medical assistants to learn the exact locales from which tumor patients came. He needed to prepare a booklet with pictures illustrating clinical, radiological, and microscopic features of the cancer. He would accept not only microscopically proven lymphomas, but also those clinically recorded cases which might not have biopsy confirmation.

Denis decided that two companions were necessary for the trip, for if one became ill, there would still be two to carry on. Dr. Ted Williams of Kuluva, the mechanical genius who could keep any car in running order, came to his mind. For the second companion, he thought of a Canadian missionary-friend, Dr. Cliff Nelson. Both agreed to go, and Denis asked Ted to have a suitable car equipped by the time he returned from his home leave.

The Burkitt family left Uganda by plane on March 17, 1961, and reached Laragh by the end of the month. But the home wasn't the same. Dick had faithfully mowed the expanses of lawn, but missing were the colorful beds of annual flowers so meticulously tended by Gwen Burkitt. The more somber perennial flowers were bravely rising above encroaching weeds. The former charm of Laragh was gone. The home place desperately missed Denis's parents who had once made it so idyllic.

While in Laragh, Denis and Olive invited some of their friends from Uganda to stay with them, taking them sightseeing to various points of beauty. Laragh, they found, was not the only place undergoing change. Sadly, Lough Erne did not hold its former attraction, or Mullaghmore, for both had become commercialized with busloads of noisy, littering tourists.

Denis left the family at Laragh to fill two scheduled engagements in London. The first invitation was to speak in the huge hall of the Royal College of Surgeons— quite an honor. But as the hour for his presentation approached, he was embarrassed to find an audience of only twelve persons in a room commodious enough for a thousand. However, John Oxenham's little saying was to prove true in time:,

> A man may count the acorns on an oak,
> But who can say
> How many great oaks may,
> From one acorn be born.

It happened that one of the twelve persons in attendance was Professor Pulvertaft, a pathologist who would one day go full time into research on the African lymphoma.

Denis's other lecture, at the Middlesex Hospital, had been publicized by a typewritten announcement on a bulletin board:

> A COMBINED MEDICAL AND SURGICAL STAFF MEETING WILL BE
> HELD ON WEDNESDAY, 22ND MARCH, 1961 AT 5:15 P.M. IN THE
> COURTAULD LECTURE THEATRE. MR. D.P. BURKITT FROM MAK-
> ERERE COLLEGE, UGANDA WILL TALK ON "THE COMMONEST

CHILDREN'S CANCER IN TROPICAL AFRICA, A HITHERTO UNREC-
OGNIZED SYNDROME."

This notice caught the eye of a young virologist, Dr. Anthony Epstein, who worked nearby in the Bland Sutton Institute. He listened attentively to the lecture and was especially impressed by its geographical distribution which suggested to him the possible involvement of a biological agent.

After the lecture, Epstein excitedly rushed up, saying, "You may have the missing piece of an important medical jigsaw puzzle. My work has involved isolating viruses from chicken cancers. It sounds like there could be a virus in your lymphoma. How can I get some pieces of fresh tumor tissue?"

Denis, equally encouraged by this energetic researcher, promised, "I can make arrangements with an airline to send you fresh tumor tissue on ice in a thermos. I believe we can work out something with BOAC (the British Overseas Air Corporation) which flies planes into Entebbe. We can send packages deliverable to you in London." Epstein promised to work with the airline on the London end.

As the young virologist left the auditorium, Epstein pulled the typewritten notice announcing the Burkitt lecture from the bulletin board to be filed away.

*****

Sorting and packing occupied much of the time at Laragh for Gwen and Jim Burkitt had rarely thrown anything away. When Denis picked up one of his father's old guns, Olive exclaimed, "Just seeing that gun reminds me of an amusing incident. Do you remember the morning we were awakened by the firing of a gun right close to us?"

"You must mean the time Daddy shot a rabbit out in his garden from his bedroom window," Denis said, laughing. "He was always a good shot."

"He must have been in his eighties then," Olive recalled. "I was surprised he would kill any living thing, he loved the birds so much."

"Yes, but he loved his garden too," Denis countered, "and he couldn't stand to see rabbits eating his precious vegetables." Looking over the gun, Denis said, "I think I'll take this gun back to Africa with me."

"Here are some of your father's letters and reports, and here's your mother's diary," Olive said. "I'm sure you'll want to go through these things carefully. No telling what you'll find." She closed the small box and retied a ribbon around it. Since they couldn't keep every precious item, it would be necessary to hold an auction. But who could watch new owners carrying away the familiar pieces?

In the midst of all the confusion at Laragh, Denis noticed an international news item in the April 11th daily paper regarding his and O'Conor's co-authored article, just published in the March issue of *Cancer*, the prestigious journal of the American

Cancer Society. It described the strange cancer of African children which Burkitt and O'Conor suggested might be caused by a virus. This first published intimation of a possible viral role in the African lymphoma was to be followed later by an overwhelming interest within the medical community.

Another meaningful event for the family took place at the old Trory church, which occupied a knoll overlooking Lough Erne, about a half-mile down the road from Laragh. On April 30, Denis, Olive and their three daughters attended a special memorial service for James and Gwendolyn Burkitt. A stone Gaelic cross marked their burial places in the Trory country churchyard. On this beautiful spring Sunday morning, the sun glinted on the mirror-like waters of the lake, reflecting in its blue surface the green islands of the opposite shore. It was a fitting day for the community's final farewell to James and Gwen Burkitt.

The church bell rang out across the countryside, announcing the service. A harmonium served for an organ and accompanied a small choir of half-a-dozen village girls and a couple of young men, who led the singing of hymns.

Denis had been asked to unveil a brass plaque on the wall above the former Burkitt pew. It read:

> To the glory of God and in loving memory of
> James Parsons Burkitt and of Gwendolyn, his
> wife, of Laragh, faithful servants of God in
> the parish for many years.

Saying goodbye forever to all the old haunts at Laragh was sad for Judy and Cassy, as the Burkitt estate had always been their magical castle. To close the door and turn the key of Laragh for the last time was painful also for Denis and Olive. Laragh would be sold after they left. This was the end of a lovely family era.

But 1961 would also be the beginning of another era for Denis P. Burkitt, M.D.

8

THE 10,000-MILE SAFARI

Eager to begin further investigation of the lymphoma tumor, Tony Epstein arrived in Kampala in July 1961, shortly after Burkitt's return to Uganda. From Epstein, Denis learned of friction between two major cancer-research foundations in England. Both of these groups were determined to get involved with the African lymphoma work. This pleased him immensely.

Dennis Wright had already been sending fresh tumor tissue on ice by air to Epstein's London laboratory. The plan worked well for him for the next several years. Not only Tony Epstein, but others were clamoring for tissue. On July 21, Burkitt recorded in his diary: "After my operations today, quite a crowd waiting for tissue from the lymphoma biopsy. There were two from New York, one from London, and of course our own people."

As Burkitt planned for his upcoming fact-finding safari, he wrote letters requesting grant money to cover the expenses. He plotted the route the team would take, figuring they would visit over fifty hospitals in twelve African countries. Most of the hospitals would be mission-operated. Denis considered them more reliable than government hospitals since their personnel changed less over the years. Writing to the directors of each of these hospitals, he gave an estimated time of their arrival and departure and explained what his team hoped to learn regarding the lymphoma, He enclosed his brochure illustrated with his photographs of typical lymphoma cases and description of clinical, x-ray and biopsy findings.

September, 1961 was a full month with several significant entries in his diary. On September 4, Denis recorded something exciting for the future: "Received letter from Joe Burchenal today offering me a trip to America. How things crowd in! Of course, I'd love to go if I could get away, though it would mean leaving Olive again."

On September 9, he wrote: "Read a paper on 'Geographical Surgery' at a special symposium in honor of my colleague who initially gave me such a hard time. He is about to leave Uganda permanently." September 13: "Letter from U.S. asking for information regarding possibility of a television program." September 17: "Olive and I saw Cassy off to school in England. We watched the twinkling lights of the airplane in the night sky till they disappeared. Judy is still attending her school in Kenya." September 20: "Passport visas and car documents required for safari, received." September 30: "Ted arrived with the car. Getting it ready for the long safari. He has various innovations for it."

Happily, Dr. Bill Davis, director of the Ugandan Medical Service, agreed to give Denis ten weeks with full pay to go on the safari. Now grant money began coming in. Sir Harold Himsworth from the Medical Research Council in London sent £ 200 ($600.00). Through Burchenal's suggestion, New York's Sloane-Kettering Institute contributed £100 ($300.00). Before long, Denis had collected about £700 ($2100.00), a pittance for most researchers, but Denis had an amazing facility for making money stretch.

Dr. Ted Williams, one of his two companions for the trip, had already arrived and was tuning up the 1954 Ford station wagon, purchased for £ 250 ($750.00) from a missionary fleeing the Congo during the Simba revolution. Ted had ordered large sheets of metal welded over the bottom of the car so that sharp rocks in the roads wouldn't puncture the gas tank. He thought to screw a steel box on the car in a hidden place, where they could keep passports and valuable documents. In addition, he chose important extra parts for emergency use and bought two spare tires, which he secured on the roof. Ted was a real asset to the team, for he had not only been born in Nairobi, but had been a missionary in Uganda for about fifteen years and spoke several African dialects.

Dr. Cliff Nelson, the other member of the safari, had been a family physician in Alberta, Canada before coming to Africa. He and his wife, Beth, had been good friends of the Burkitts since their arrival in Uganda in 1958. Nelson had left Canada originally to work for the colonial service of Uganda. but recently he had resigned from the government and joined the African Inland Mission in Western Tanzania.

When the loaded Ford station wagon left Kampala the morning of October 7, 1961, it was no wonder Denis felt exhilarated. Everything was coming together satisfactorily. He and Ted were to meet Cliff en route in a few days. Little did they dream that their journey would have repercussions around the world. Denis later stated, "We were conscious only that each of us was in Africa as a result of God's leading, and that for all we have, we are indebted to Him."

Denis had marked the course of their trip, town by town, on a map. He took along his typewriter to record data and interesting happenings along the way, intending to post these in letters to Olive back home. At about 9 a.m., they left Kampala and traveled the first eighty-six miles to Masaka on a tarmac road surrounded by monotonous country with low hills. Beyond Masaka the good road ended. They passed through plantations of eucalyptus and stopped for a picnic lunch which Olive had prepared. "This is better than a ten-course lunch at the Imperial Hotel in Kampala!" Denis said appreciatively, for in his eyes, Olive's food could never be improved upon. Ted, munching on a sandwich, had to agree.

Arriving in Bukoba on Lake Victoria's west shore, they found a small hotel and then looked up the District Medical Officer. On entering the house of this officer, an Indian doctor, they were surprised to find a text framed on the wall.

Christ is the Head of this House,
the Unseen Guest at Every Meal,
the Silent Listener
to Every Conversation.

As they went through the medical questionnaire with this Christian physician, they learned that his was the only government hospital for a population of 600,000. And yes, many cases of the lymphoma occurred along the shores of Lake Victoria.

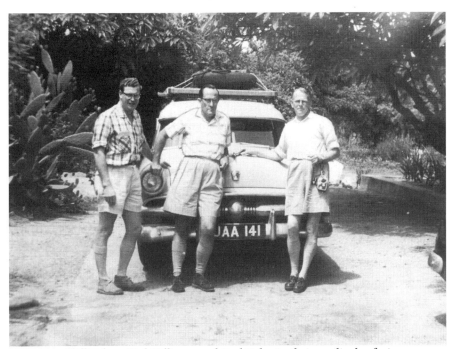

Cliff Nelson, Ted Williams and Burkitt begin their medical safari.

Later, leaving the lake behind, the station wagon climbed 1,000 feet to Ndolage and a Swedish Mission Hospital. Although now but thirty miles from Lake Victoria, they found that the tumor was never seen on this plateau. Many of the hospital's patients came from the more mountainous areas across the nearby Rwanda border. After spending the nights of October 8 and 9 as guests of the missionaries there, Denis and Ted returned to the lake and turned south. Cliff Nelson and family were driving toward them on the same road. When they met, the group had a picnic lunch, following which, Beth and her children drove on to Kampala to spend the time while their husbands were gone with Olive.

October 11 found the heavily-burdened station wagon jouncing along for about 200 miles through endless, dusty bush, rarely meeting another vehicle. As is often the case with doctors, the conversation of the car's three occupants soon turned to interesting medical cases.

Ted began, asking, "Have either of you ever delivered triplets?" Of course they hadn't. He continued his story, "Many years ago, a woman came to have her baby at Kuluva. Instead of one, she had three—all in a hurry. Two of our overseas nurses, who had only recently arrived in Africa, undertook the care of the three tiny babies in their own house," Ted explained. "As it turned out, the caring included guarding the babies! Twins are traditionally an evil omen in our area, but triplets were even worse!

"Relatives tried to snatch away the babies for the next six weeks, if you can imagine, but the parents were most grateful to the nurses for saving their babies' lives." Ted was now reaching the climax of his narration. "Since the hospital staff, at that time, had a vacancy, the father was given training as a nurse. He became a Christian and is now the head of the nursing staff. The three little girls have recently reached their twelfth birthdays."

"That tale is hard to beat," Denis admitted, "but listen to this one. We have many trauma cases at Mulago, some of them really strange. But I think this case tops the list. One morning an African came into my clinic complaining of headache. When I examined him, I noticed a three-inch scar under his left jaw. I asked what had caused the injury, to which the man replied, 'Oh, I was standing near where a friend was mowing the lawn one day and suddenly noticed I was bleeding on the neck.' " Denis asked, "Would you like to guess what I found?"

"I haven't a clue," Cliff said.

"Must have been something terribly unusual to improve upon my story," Ted said, with a smile.

"When we took an x-ray of the man's skull," Denis said, "we found a small, triangular-shaped blade from the lawn mower in the middle of his head! How it ever got there without severing vital arteries, veins and nerves, no one could comprehend."

"You've topped me!" Ted said, "Amazing!"

All three were silent for a while as the boring road stretched endlessly on. Denis suddenly broke the silence with a profound observation. "This must be the safest safari to ever go through Africa. Here we are, three doctors, each loaded with a huge box of medications for every eventuality, and we're continually making a bee line from one hospital to the next."

"How true!" Cliff remarked. "I'm thinking of the medical pioneer, Dr. Albert Cook and his wife, Kathryn. If they could have envisioned us, wouldn't they have considered us 'softies?' "

"Yes, but, at the same time, I'll wager they'd have envied us a bit!" Ted added.

North of Lake Tanganyika, the trio climbed thirty miles through scenic hills to a Seventh-day Adventist Hospital. Here they met missionaries from South Africa who were most helpful but reported no tumors in their area. The road descending from this hospital to Kigoma was treacherous. Some sections of the narrow road, carved out of the mountain, had a sheer drop-off. Ted, driving at this point punned, "I have a 'Cliff' on both sides of me!" Before reaching Kigoma they descended 3,000 feet. En route at Ujiji, they stood under the historic mango tree where Stanley and Livingston met on November 10, 1871. Denis figured his father had been fifteen months old at the time.

A few miles farther, they arrived in Kigoma, where they found the town's one hotel reasonably cheap. Denis appeared, to the other two men, visibly relieved when he learned that the hotel had no rooms with baths. "I don't mind economizing in every way possible," he commented to his two companions. "If I couldn't walk a few steps down the hall to the washroom, I'd feel I was growing decadent."

They registered there for the night before meeting the District Medical Officer, who advised them that the lymphoma was prevalent in this low-lying country northeast of Lake Tanganyika. The following day, they left Kigoma early and traveled 250 miles on a dry, dusty road, scarcely meeting a vehicle or a single soul. This gave them time to theorize on their findings thus far.

"Even though we've scarcely begun the trip," Denis began, "has anything impressed either of you?"

After giving it some thought, Ted, who had done most of the driving, observed, "We've been up and down a lot of mountains. There were no tumor patients in the mountains at Ndolage nor at the Seventh-day Adventist Hospital on the edge of Rwanda."

"That's right," Denis said, as he matched Ted's statement with notations on his map. "However, the medical officers at Bukoba on Lake Victoria and at Kigoma near Lake Tanganyika reported many cases."

"I wonder if altitude might be a factor in the incidence of the disease," Cliff proposed. "But if so, why?" he questioned.

Denis pondered the problem. "Several researchers, of course, including myself, are already thinking in terms of a possible viral cause of the tumor to account for the geographic distribution. But why should a virus be affected by altitude?" He wound down a window for a breath of fresh air, but quickly raised it again as dust poured into the car.

They were driving through a desolate part of Africa, dry, hot and inhospitable, when the car came to a hesitating stop. The engine had been coughing occasionally, giving Ted time to think of a remedy if needed. As the engine died, he hopped out of the car and, after digging for a piece of wire in a tool box on the back seat, used the wire to connect the battery directly to the coil. He climbed back into the station wagon and pushed the starter. The motor began purring again—much to their relief. "That's why I invited Ted on the trip!" Denis said. "He treats mechanical problems as if they were child's play."

To dispel the monotony of driving, they sometimes sang songs from Cliff's hymn book. An occasional antelope or giraffe added momentary excitement. Denis often thought, *how fortunate that Ted welded that extra sheet of metal to the car's under parts*, for frequently the vehicle scraped the high middle ridge of the road. When they stopped to fill their drinking cups from a four-gallon plastic water container, they wondered what the people in the area did for water. They hadn't encountered a lake, pond or stream in many miles.

Finally, as they entered Sumbawanga, they were struck with the beauty of the lavender-flowered jacaranda trees lining the dusty roads. They spent a night in the rest house before proceeding into Northern Rhodesia (Zambia). In talking with the Medical Officer in Abercorn, they found that, despite being in the lowlands at the southern tip of Lake Tanganyika, there was no evidence of the tumor in this dry, dusty area.

As they traveled on, their conversation naturally came back to their findings of the previous day. The dry, "tumorless" area they had just passed through shot holes in their theory. Low-lying, parched lake shores were not a sure place to find the tumor. "At least we're making valid observations," Denis reminded them. "If we hadn't taken this trip, we might have been inclined to make false assumptions. We'll have to record this area at the southern end of Lake Tanganyika as an exception, that is, if the pattern we first observed proves true."

On and on they journeyed, hundreds of miles through dry, barren lands, finding no tumor at several hospitals. To break the monotony, Ted began discussing the Flying Doctor Services of East Africa. The organization's surgeon and founder, Dr. Michael Wood, had flown into Kuluva to help out on several occasions. "One time I had a patient with severe abdominal pain, and x-rays revealed a huge stone in a kidney. Dr. Wood performed the surgery and removed the stone."

"A kidney stone?" Denis could hardly believe it. "I've never seen a kidney stone at Mulago." But Ted verified the finding, admitting that he, himself, had never seen a kidney stone in an African before. "That's why I needed surgical assistance. At Kuluva, we have a radio call set and can get in instant contact with the Flying Doctor's control room in Nairobi to ask for advice or help in emergencies, such as in this case."

"It's really a wonderful service," Cliff agreed, for he too knew what it was like to be isolated with a complicated surgical emergency.

After driving beyond their 2,000-mile mark, the team reached a hospital near Tunduma. It was run by a lady doctor, over eighty, like Denis a graduate of Trinity College, Dublin. She had seen but one case of the tumor; it was in a patient from the upper Luangwa Valley. Proceeding to high, dry Northern Zambia, they found no tumors, but on descending to the Karonga hospital on the western shores of Lake Nyasa, they found many.

Unpaved roads led through continually changing terrain, up over mountains and down into valleys. One of their most precarious roads was the climb from Karonga to Livingstonia, which ascended over 2,000 feet in seven miles but represented only about two miles distance in a straight line. Denis counted 112 bends and 22 hairpin turns with such steep grades that the car could barely maneuver in the lowest gear. The engine boiled repeatedly, requiring the addition of more water. At the summit, on the Malawi plateau, they found no report of the tumor in the local hospital.

Driving along this high plateau through Mzuzu to Mzimba, they found an African doctor who said quite emphatically that there was no lymphoma in his area. In Mzimba, they met a missionary couple with Irish accents. Denis, of course was curious to know where they'd come from. "A place called Enniskillen in North Ireland," was the reply.

"Unbelievable! That's my home town!" Denis exclaimed; but he couldn't remember having seen them before. "Denis Burkitt," he introduced himself. Upon learning his name, they asked if he might be a son of J.P. Burkitt. Denis was nonplused to find persons in the middle of Africa who had known his father!

Their journey next took them through the Nyasaland highlands (Malawi), where there was no trace of the lymphoma. But as they again entered the low-lying areas around Blantyre, the capital of Malawi, the tumor reappeared.

From Blantyre, they must cross the Zambezi River near the southern end of Malawi. Since it had been terribly dry and the river was unusually low, the ferry wasn't running. Consequently, they had to change their plans and detour about 150 miles on mere tracks in the bush to put the car on a goods train and cross the river by the longest railway bridge in Africa. Arriving at the place to load the car at 3:30 in the afternoon, they learned that the train wasn't due until 9 p.m. The blistering heat

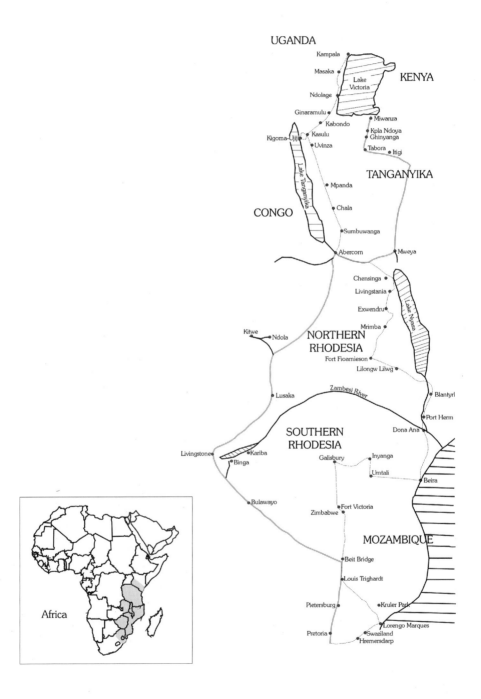

October—November, 1961
Safari route from Kampala, Uganda to Johannesberg, South Africa.

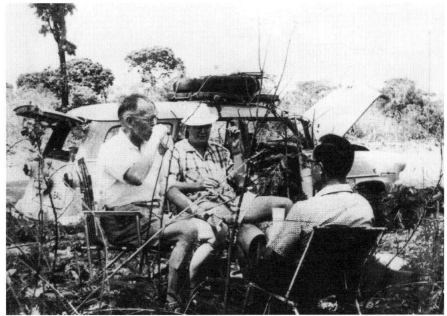

Time out for cooling off the car and lunch-break.

bore down on them for there was no shade, and worse than that, they had nothing to do.

Even after they had the station wagon lifted onto a flat car, they still had to wait for the train to take them across the two-and-a-half-mile-long bridge. At dusk the mosquitoes descended, forcing the men to choose between sitting inside their oven-like car or being unmercifully bitten outside. They alternately tried both. Unloading the station wagon from the flat car took an additional two hours. By then it was midnight. Since there was no lodging accommodation, they had no alternative but to travel on in the dark toward Beira.

However, they soon found their road had again become a mere track and were thankful for the compass they had brought along. After many tedious and anxious miles, they at length spotted a twinkling light in the distance and came upon an open telegraph office. The operator gave them directions to the capital city, so they continued to drive all through the night. At last, they reached a good road and pulled into Beira in Mozambique by breakfast time.

Contact with the local hospitals in Beira confirmed their suspicion that the lymphoma would be found along the entire Mozambique coast. They traveled inland over miles of good tarmac road, gained altitude through green countryside and mists, and reached another hospital at 2,000 feet elevation. As expected, they found no tumors. Their journey next took them through Zimbabwe's beautiful mountains with superb vistas, on good roads. The afternoon of November 3 they reached

Salisbury (now Harare) with its lovely houses, well-kept lawns, flowering jacaranda and bougainvillea. Their group was treated royally and given tours of hospitals and surrounding points of interest. But no lymphoma was known there.

By far the most interesting stop of their entire trip was at Lourenço Marques in southern Mozambique. In this Portuguese colony they contacted Dr. Prates, pathologist in a large hospital. Denis had corresponded with him earlier and knew that his main interest was liver cancer, for this city had the highest incidence of liver cancer in the world. When they made rounds on the hospital wards, they noted two or three children, both black and white, together occupying single beds.

Dr. Prates, they soon learned, had developed a custom of having postmortem plaster casts made of his most bizarre cases. When Denis showed him the lymphoma brochure, he went to his museum shelves and pulled out cast after cast of children's heads with grotesquely distorted faces and jaws—the African lymphoma! The three men excitedly carried the casts up to the hospital roof and took pictures of the lineup as a visible demonstration of the tumor's occurrence in that part of Africa.

In addition, Prates spread out for examination his past five years' records of all children's cancers. Denis found over forty cases of the tumor in this city and recorded the patient's addresses for later plotting on his map.

Lourenço Marques was the most southerly place reporting the tumor. Inland, in mountainous Swaziland, they stopped at a very fine 250-bed Nazarene Hospital in Manzini. The doctors were most cordial, as well as positive that they had never seen the tumor.

When they reached South Africa, they found that it resembled any modern European country, with heavy traffic in town after town. In Johannesburg they headed for the South African Institute for Medical Research, where a prearranged meeting with Dr. Oettle was to take place. All the surgery professors from the South African medical schools were meeting simultaneously with the team's visit.

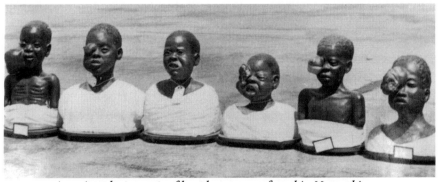

Amazing plaster casts of lymphoma cases found in Mozambique.

During the question and comment period after Burkitt's lecture, there was general feeling that he had made an outstanding contribution. How could he help being pleased and excited as a groundswell of medical opinion backed his theory? At home he'd had some opposition to his views, but now thousands of miles away from Kampala in South Africa, medical opinion and enthusiasm were swinging to his side. It was a heady moment.

On the South African elevated plateau where Dr. Oettle had told him earlier there was no lymphoma, he now learned they had recently found a case, a European child. Although the child lived in Johannesburg, he had been to lower altitudes for holidays. Otherwise, only along the northern coast of Natal adjacent to Mozambique had any cases of the tumor been found.

Now the team began their return trip. They found no tumors reported in Pietersburg. It was present in the valleys of the Zambezi and Limpopo rivers but not in the hill country between the rivers. By the time the three men reached Zambia, torrential rains had begun, the worst in a hundred years.

Returning through Tanzania, they planned to stop at Cliff's hospital in Kola Ndota, near Shinyanga. However, they found a swollen stream running across the road and could proceed no farther. They spent the night stretched on top of the luggage in the car, alternately fighting mosquitoes when the windows were open and sweltering when the windows were closed. By morning the floods had subsided enough for them to pass through and drive on to Cliff's hospital at Kola Ndota. Here

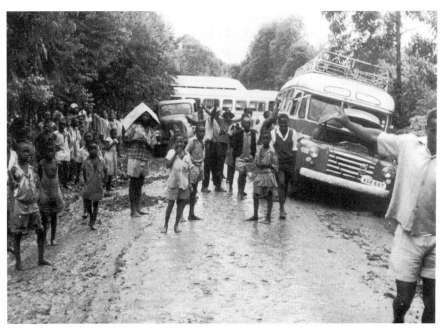

Torrential rain and muddy roads bogged-down vehicles.

they learned that further travel was nearly impossible because of flooded bridges and washed-out roads. They would have to postpone their prospective trip through Rwanda and Burundi.

Because of the heavy rains and swollen river, they turned back, put the car on a goods train, and boarded it themselves. They elected to head for a port on the south shore of Lake Victoria where the car was lifted by crane onto a ship to cross the lake. When they reached Mwanza, a port on the east shore of the lake, they had the car taken off the ship.

A several hour wait near Kisuma held them up while cars and buses, lying on their sides blocking the road, were removed. They had one more hospital to visit. After it, and two more days' driving through deep mud and flooded roads, their trip ended at Mulago to a "Welcome Home" banner, and confetti showers from three waiting wives and their children.

Only a frugal Irishman could have organized this 10,000-mile, ten-week safari, visiting fifty-seven hospitals in eight countries, at a cost—after selling the car for £125—of only £678 ($2034.00). An inexpensive research project indeed! But what valuable pieces had they found to fit into the lymphoma jigsaw puzzle?

9

FILLING IN THE GAPS

At the Mulago Hospital in Kampala, news spread that the lymphoma was "altitude-dependent." This jaw tumor, limited to childhood and geographically confined to a central belt across Africa, seemed to be getting more unusual the more it was studied. Burkitt, convinced by now that some virus must be involved, began thinking of a possible insect carrier. He needed to consult with an entomologist familiar with African insect distribution, so he looked up Dr. Alex Haddow, director of the East African Virus Research Institute in Entebbe.

Haddow studied Burkitt's map, newly revised after the long safari. He concluded, with some authority, "It's true that you've not found the tumor at higher altitudes. I can see that from your notes. I also see that the altitude barrier varies with the latitude. The tumor apparently stops at five thousand feet altitude at the equator; at about three thousand feet, a thousand miles south of the equator; and at only a few hundred feet altitude, two thousand miles below the equator." The team had gathered enough evidence to support this. Haddow paused, then added, "But I don't think 'altitude' is the factor."

Surprised, Burkitt asked, "If not altitude, what else could it be?"

Haddow answered, "I think you have a **temperature barrier**." He pointed on the map to various mountain ranges over which Denis's team had traveled and explained, "The temperature at these higher altitudes often falls below sixty degrees Fahrenheit, depending upon the distance from the equator."

Burkitt asked, "Just what do you have in mind? " He had his own ideas but wanted to see what his friend would say. Haddow reached for a book on the shelf and reminded Denis, "Some insects don't survive with prolonged low temperatures—mosquitoes for example."

This was what Burkitt wanted to hear. He folded his map. Had Haddow intimated that an insect vector carrying an infectious agent, such as a virus, was the cause of the tumor? Denis told him that this same idea had come to the minds of many researchers when they first considered the strange geographic distribution. He crossed his arms over his chest. But he had to tell Haddow the one discordant finding made on the trip.

"Even though the tumor was common in nearly every low-lying place we visited," Burkitt said, "there was one hot, low area where we found absolutely no tumors. This puzzled us and almost shot our 'altitude theory.' What does this finding do to a 'temperature barrier' theory?"

"Denis," Haddow concluded, "it's obvious you don't have all the facts yet."

This parting comment precipitated Denis's plans for a second, then a third fact-finding safari to bring together all information possible. Because of the heavy rains and flooding they had been unable to visit Rwanda and Burundi. A trip then to those countries became a "must" which had to be squeezed into his schedule at the first opportunity.

*****

As a result of the widely-read article appearing in the March 1961 *Cancer* journal, the international news media besieged Kampala, the Mulago Hospital, and especially Denis Burkitt. Jack Darling described the scene: "The publication made Kampala a honey pot attracting the bees of cancer research and virology from all over the world."

On January 24, 1962, Denis made a note in his diary: "American journalists are taking photos and asking questions. The photographers join me on ward rounds." On February 6 he recorded: "U.S. television team here. The girls thought this great fun. Spent three-and-a-half hours for possibly three-and-a-half minutes television time. Ian hated it." Subsequently, articles about the African tumor, the long safari, and the possible virus implication appeared in *Time* and *Reader's Digest*.

At the end of March, 1962, Tony Epstein came out to Uganda a second time with a plan to inject monkeys. Burkitt accompanied him early one morning on a motor launch in Lake Victoria, going to several islands. At an island about ten miles out in the lake, they made a foray into the jungle to find African trappers from whom they could buy monkeys for his proposed experiments. The Africans bargained to collect several suckling African green monkeys with their nursing mothers.

It was getting late in the afternoon when Denis hired a motorized dugout canoe for their return trip. They had just left the island, when the motor sputtered and stopped. The African boatman restarted the reluctant motor, but it operated for only a short time. Repeatedly this nerve-racking cycle continued as night came on. Several worry-filled hours in total darkness passed until the boat at last pulled into its intended destination.

For the monkey experiment, Burkitt removed tumor tissue from a five-year-old girl with a typical jaw lymphoma. Epstein prepared a special tumor suspension and inoculated it into the peritoneal cavities of four infant monkeys, which were then kept with their mothers for observation at the East African Virus Research Institute in Entebbe.

*****

As various renowned medical personages from England, Canada, and the United States visited Kampala, Denis had the opportunity of meeting many medical "experts." With so much continued excitement over the lymphoma, he considered making a documentary medical film, since not everyone interested in the tumor could make the trip to Uganda. Working on this project was just one more distraction to add to his already busy schedule.

Finally, about the middle of April, he arranged a flight with the East Africa Medical Research Foundation for a trip to both of the mountainous, populous countries of Burundi and Rwanda. When the well-known virologist, Dr. Gilbert Dalldorf, then with an American team in Nairobi, learned of Burkitt's projected trip, he asked to accompany him. Dalldorf, also interested in the African lymphoma, had years earlier stated that any proved causal relationship between a virus and human cancer would have tremendous impact on cancer research. He now firmly believed that this African lymphoma was the tumor that might lead to just such a discovery.

As the two men were piloted in the small plane, Denis pointed out the west coast of Lake Victoria, the volcanic peaks of northern Rwanda, some as high as 11,000 feet, and then in the distance, Lake Tanganyika. They were looking down on the Nile-Congo watershed, one of the most densely populated areas in all Africa.

Their first destination in the extreme south of Burundi was the capital city, Bujumbura, located at the northern end of Lake Tanganyika, and about 3,000 feet above sea level. Here they visited the well-established Bujumbura medical school, operated by Belgian doctors who spoke some English. Nearly all the patients coming to this hospital were from the northern hills. In spite of inquiries, and examination of surgical and pathology records, they could find no evidence of the tumor, with the exception of a single case from the plains.

The next day they flew on to Kigali, the capital of Rwanda, where again they conferred with several doctors, in both government and mission hospitals. Some of the doctors had been practicing there for over twenty-five years. None had seen the tumor in that hilly population, in spite of having been alerted to the tumor for the previous three years. Burkitt and Dalldorf returned that evening to Nairobi, having accomplished in two days what would have taken over a week by car. There was one disadvantage Denis observed. The quick flights precluded the possibility of the kind of extended discussion and speculation which he had enjoyed on the long safari with Ted and Cliff.

*****

In spite of his busy medical involvement, Denis never neglected his spiritual commitments. Occasionally, he took time for Bible study with prisoners. The attendance at their meetings varied from seventy to twice that number. Olive also had her outside interests and worked with a youthful group called the Crusader Girls. In addition, they often had large groups for Bible study in their home. Denis rarely allowed pure busyness to crowd out these appointments.

As the weeks and months passed, one question kept coming to Burkitt's mind. Was this African lymphoma a new entity, or had it just been overlooked for a long time? He leaned toward this latter idea, for had he not found identical cases in old hospital records?

One day while searching through re-

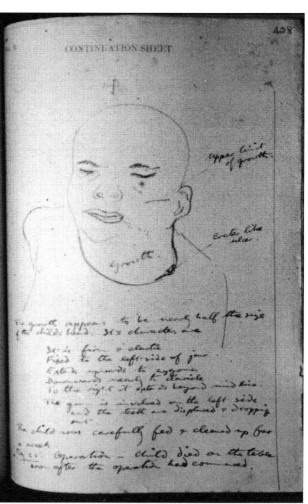

Drawing from Dr. Albert Cook's notebook showing child with a jaw tumor.

cords from the Mengo Hospital where two of his daughters had been born, Denis came upon evidence which clarified the question. Mengo Mission Hospital, the oldest in East Africa, had been founded in 1897 by the famous Dr., later Sir, Albert Cook. Cook had kept excellent clinical notes and often supplemented them with sketches. Among Cook's records, Denis found a drawing of a child with jaw swellings recognizable as the same cancer he was investigating. He had answered the question. He was researching not a new, but a hitherto neither named nor understood disease.

Only recently Denis had acquired a copy of the new biography of Dr. Cook, *That Good Physician*, by Brian O'Brien. He pulled this book from his office bookcase and opened it to the large map of Uganda inside the front cover. There, crisscrossing bold red lines depicted the many long medical safaris taken by the doctor, often accompanied by his wife, Katherine. *Our long safari was luxurious compared with this one the Cooks took in 1900*, thought Denis, as he scanned O'Brien's descriptive text:

On April 15th the safari left Namirembe [near Kampala where the Mengo Hospital was located], the doctor on his ramshackle bicycle, Katherine regal on a mule and, trailing behind them, thirty porters and two cows.

The rains greeted them; the first day was a sodden wading through flooded paths over steep, slimy hills to Ndeje. Dr. Cook's bicycle collapsed so many times, shedding spokes every mile or so, that he sent it back as more dangerous than useful. From then until his return he walked…. Seven hundred reported for treatment and six operations were performed amid shouts of wonder….

Wading, fighting off mosquitoes, floundering through swamps, they reached the Kafu River, over a mile wide. The only means of crossing was a palm stem with the pith scraped out.

A plague of hornets scattered the porters and had to be driven off with blazing grass. Finally the rapid stream was crossed; but the missionaries were without food from dawn until late night, when they were informed that the dugout had capsized with the food and surgical boxes in it.

Wearily they opened the case and spent most of the night carefully drying the instruments and smearing them with Vaseline. When that was over they just fell into their cots, too tired to eat.

Up at 3 a.m. they were off again, climbing the slow hills of Unyoro. It was unbearably hot and humid as they crossed the plains. The only danger was from occasional elephants and a rather alarming pride of lions....

Denis could hardly believe the courage of these hardy pioneers as he read on, greatly intrigued:

> Over a hundred patients were seen at every halt. Then the going turned bad. They crossed foaming torrents over slimy tree trunks, struggled for hours through ten-foot elephant grass that soaked them to the skin, and climbed, hand under hand, down a 2,000-foot canyon to cross the Nkusi River.
>
> Passing over what looked like a shallow pool Katherine's mule sank to its girths. She rolled clear and immediately disappeared in the black slime. Dr. Cook reached desperately and dragged her to solid ground.....

What heroism! thought Denis. *And this is the man who was also a scientist. When they first came to Uganda, little was known about tropical diseases. The mosquito had not yet been proved the carrier of malaria. Cook made some important medical discoveries.* Denis read again regarding the doctor's first discovery:

> His microscope was an ancient and battered model of limited magnification.... Nevertheless, he had taken blood samples of serious cases of a special kind of fever and, examining them under the highest power of his microscope, found what he thought to be flagellated malarial parasites. He made diagrams and sent them to London with his thesis for the M.D. degree.
>
> Some time later he received a copy of the journal in which his thesis was published and a sarcastic letter from a London research scientist calling attention to the fact that this "missionary who calls himself a doctor," had offered pictures that could not be those of malarial parasites, though he did not suggest any other diagnosis. Dr. Cook, without making excuses for his makeshift apparatus, and congratulating the scornful one on his acumen, made further experiments and finally identified the parasites as the spirilla that cause relapsing fever and that they are carried by ticks. This

discovery established Dr. Cook as a research scientist to be considered with respect.

Denis could see by Cook's drawing of the child with the jaw tumor that he had not only been an astute observer but also a careful scientist, recording his findings by both word and picture. *What a privilege,* he thought, *to follow in this brilliant, godly man's footsteps! Hopefully, we can eventually add not only a diagnosis, but the cause of the tumor depicted in Dr. Cook's little sketch.*

*****

Anxious now to add a West Africa geographical study to his East Africa data, Burkitt on May 15, was off to the Congo, this time by a commercial airline. Looking down at the terrain with its sparsity of mountains, he noted how the topography of West and East Africa differed.

His first stop was Leopoldville, now Kinshasa, in the newly independent Zaire. Everywhere he saw evidence of the recent Simba revolution. There was an atmosphere of suspicion in the air. No sooner had Denis landed than his passport was confiscated, which didn't add to his feeling of security. Fortunately, an English-trained Indian surgeon, Dr. Jain, met him on arrival and immediately tried to help him find his passport; however, it had completely disappeared. Only with the intervention of the Louvanium University administration were they able to find it, after going from office to office in the city. Thus Denis's first day in Kinshasa was a scientific waste.

The following day, Dr. Jain introduced Denis to Belgian physicians at the university who were able to supply him with the information he sought. Although they commonly saw the lymphoma in the university hospital, all the patients had been referred from outside the city, an observation he noted carefully. He visited a major mission hospital in Kimpese, where the lymphoma was also seen. After several days, he was relieved to depart from chaotic Kinshasa.

His next stop was Lagos, Nigeria. Officials from the Ministry of Health met him and provided lodging in a hotel, luxurious by East African standards. The next morning he was off to Port Harcourt in the Niger Delta. Doctors in the government hospital of this small, steamy town readily recognized the syndrome when shown Denis's photographs. On returning to Lagos, Burkitt met Will Davey, Professor of Surgery and an acquaintance, who drove him a hundred miles northeast of Lagos to Ibadan University. This was one of the best-known medical schools in tropical Africa. In later years, doctors there would make notable contributions to the treatment of the African lymphoma.

Burkitt lectured on the disease at the university. Afterward, he learned that the tumor had only recently, through his own work, been recognized as the commonest childhood cancer in southern Nigeria. Professor Davey drove him for interviews to other area hospitals, where he learned further of the local prevalence of the lymphoma.

From Ibadan, Denis chose to take the next leg of his journey, to northern Kano, by train. At eye level, he felt better able to evaluate the terrain. The farther he traveled on the 400-mile trip to Kano, the drier the land became, a marked contrast to humid, tropical Ibadan and Lagos. Kano was almost a desert, hot and desiccating. He could feel his hands and lips becoming chapped. Even the dress of the people was different—long, loose gowns rather than the Westernized garb in southern Nigeria. In Kano, Denis interviewed several doctors at the large city hospital, built to accommodate the health needs of the population of 3,000,000 people within a 30-mile radius. With repeated inquiries, augmented by his pictures of lymphoma cases, he could obtain no positive identification of the lymphoma. No cancers of this type were known in the area.

This is interesting, thought Denis. *In spite of Kano's being at a low elevation, there is no lymphoma.* Then his mind went back to a similar stretch of land on their long safari. *That dry, dusty, hot drive between Kigoma and Sumbawanga in Tanzania, west of Lake Tanganyiga. We thought when we heard there was no tumor in that area that our "altitude theory" was shot. It was low land, just like this—and it was also almost a desert like Kano. Maybe, as Haddow suggested, there is another factor besides a "temperature barrier" dependent upon the altitude.*

From Kano, he resorted to air travel again and flew to Jos, the only mountain plateau in Western Nigeria. Stay-

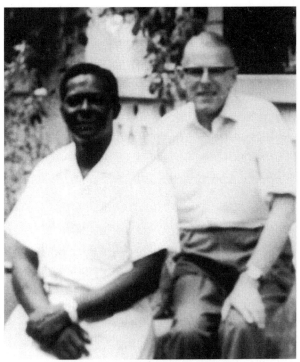

Denis with Dr. Cofie George in Accra.

ing in a large mission hospital there, he learned that, as expected, there was no lymphoma among the population of the cool plateau. However, the tumor did occur in the surrounding tropical plains.

At the coastal city of Accra, the capital of Ghana, he met his old friend and classmate from Trinity College, Dr. Cofie George. This African had inspired Denis twenty-five years earlier to consider medical service in Africa. *Just think*, Denis contemplated, *what if the Colonial Medical Service had accepted my first application and I had come to West Africa? Would I have had the opportunity which Mulago Hospital has afforded me to study this disease? How disappointed I was at that time! God had His plan.* Denis thought once more of his dear mother's favorite proverb: **Disappointment, His Appointment. Change one letter, now I see.** Yes, God had surely had an "appointment" for him. How very good God had been to him through all these fruitful years!

He recalled the professor who had once visited Mulago from West Africa and said, "We're told that you chaps here get on with each other, but at my university, none of us do. If someone gets a new idea, he locks it up in his drawer so no one else hears about it. What's your secret?"

Burkitt had simply answered, "I suppose we get on because when anyone gets an idea, we spread it out on the table and we all sit around and talk about it." Again, as Denis thought about Providence leading him to East Africa, he thanked God for his earlier disappointment.

Burkitt remembered that he had asked this same professor if he had ever seen a case of the lymphoma in West Africa. His answer had been spoken with certainty. "I've been there a long time and I've never seen a case. I'm convinced it doesn't occur in West Africa at all."

Burkitt had told the professor, "You might be interested to know that doubtless I saw cases at Lira and Kampala before I recognized this tumor was something different. I've come to believe one has to be looking for something before one actually sees it. If you're *looking* for something and still don't see it, it's probably not there," Denis emphasized.

Interestingly, two weeks after the professor had returned to West Africa, he had written to Denis saying he had now seen his first three cases of the childhood lymphoma!

Cofie George was at the airport to meet Denis, and soon introduced his wife, Sylvia, the daughter of Sir Emmanuel Quist, speaker of the first parliament following independence, when the Gold Coast became Ghana. True to custom, Cofie and his wife showered Denis with gifts for himself and Olive. As Cofie subsequently introduced him to various medical officers, Denis learned an additional important piece of information. Although the tumor was common in southern Ghana, no cases had been reported among residents of Accra itself. *This is similar to Leopoldville,* (now

Kinshasa), thought Denis to himself. *Why is it that these two large cities are free from the disease?*

From Accra on the Gulf of Guinea, Denis flew north to Kumasi, where an old friend from his hometown, Enniskillen, cordially greeted him. Dr. Charles Boseman had preceded him through Trinity College and had been a house-surgeon in Enniskillen when Denis was a medical student. For years now, Boseman had been the most senior, well-respected surgeon in all of Ghana. He had written a textbook, *Surgery and Pathology in Africa*, and so was more than qualified to give Denis information he asked for. Boseman assured him that the tumor did indeed occur in his part of Ghana.

Denis had found this trip to West Africa most worthwhile. There were still puzzles, but hopefully he could solve them. Before flying home, he stopped at a shop and bought several school atlases listing climate, vegetation, and population densities of the various West African countries. On his return flight to Uganda, he thumbed through these books, looking for the information he needed.

In Nigeria the tumor was the commonest cancer of childhood in the warm and most southern regions of the country, but was virtually unknown in the arid plains of the north. Let's see. The rainfall of southern Nigeria is often over 200 inches a year. He ran his finger down the column in the book. *In the north, the rainfall is less than twenty inches. Quite a contrast!* Denis consulted the average temperatures of the two districts. *Hmm, the temperatures are comparable. I think we have that **other factor —it's rainfall of twenty inches or less!*** He also found an explanation for the lack of the lymphoma in Accra. Even though the surrounding areas of Ghana had heavy rainfall, Accra, in a "rain shadow," had less than twenty inches.

Thinking back to the long safari, he recalled again what they had been at a loss to explain. *The low rainfall in the hot, dry area of East Africa we passed through might account for the lack of the tumor there.* **So there are two "barriers" to prevent the occurrence of the lymphoma: temperature of less than sixty degrees Fahrenheit and rainfall of twenty inches or less.** *The next step is to find what factors in the causation of the tumor are dependent on high temperature and high rainfall. I must meet with Haddow again when I reach home.*

Haddow, as an entomologist, had immediately appreciated that the temperature-dependence of the tumor implicated some living organism. Both he and Burkitt thought most likely an insect had a part to play in transmitting a microbe, probably a cancer-causing virus.

Displaying his newest map, including both the East and the West Africa tumor distribution, Denis spoke with even greater rapidity than usual, saying, "This last trip to West Africa has been most worthwhile. I believe I've found that missing factor you wanted. The other 'barrier' is rainfall of less than twenty inches. I found that in spite of blistering heat in the dry, arid areas, there was simply no tumor." Expectantly, he asked Haddow, "What do you make of this?"

What could he make of it? Haddow took a large map of Africa and laid it out on his desk. Then he took a piece of soft yellow chalk from his desk. He next shaded in the areas where the rainfall was over twenty inches a year. He did this by referring to rainfall charts. Then he also shaded in the places where the temperature was constantly above sixty degrees. Now he was ready to compare his map with Denis's.

They held them side by side. They were closely comparable.

Next they compared their maps with the distribution maps of various diseases. Haddow pulled out maps of "sleeping sickness" (trypanosomiasis, a parasitic disease transmitted by bites of the tsetse fly); yellow fever, a viral disease, transmitted by a mosquito; and o'nyong nyong fever, meaning "pain in the bones," a new disease investigated in 1959 by Haddow's research institute, also a viral disease transmitted by a mosquito. Every one of these diseases had distribution patterns similar to that of the childhood lymphoma.

"The conclusion is pretty obvious, isn't it?" Haddow looked at Burkitt. "It certainly looks like some insect is responsible for inoculating these children with a cancer-causing agent. Of course, the only microbes thought to cause cancer, which are also known to be transmitted by insects, are viruses."

Denis picked up his map and carefully folded it. "It surely looks like we've taken one more step in confirming the suspicions we've had all along," he said, with a note of triumph in his voice.

Denis had come to the conclusion in his own mind that the lymphoma was a mosquito-borne disease. But in this he would be proven wrong.

10

THE GREAT VIRUS RACE

Virologists, other than Tony Epstein in London, joined the race to find a possible virus in the African lymphoma. In Nairobi, Dr. Gilbert Dalldorf, who accompanied Burkitt to Rwanda and Burundi, had set up a team from New York's Sloane-Kettering Institute. In England there had been disagreement between two major research institutes as to which one should go to Africa and investigate the children's strange tumor.

When news reached the British scientists that the Americans had already arrived in Nairobi, Dr. Bob Harris from the Imperial Cancer Research Foundation, through fortuitous contacts with the Royal Air Force, had his equipment flown to Entebbe. There he set up the East African Virus Research Institute. The pathologists at Kampala began supplying fresh lymphoma tumor tissue not only to Epstein in London, but also to Dalldorf in Nairobi and to Harris in Entebbe. Virus laboratories in Sweden, Japan and other places also put in their requests.

For more than seventy-five years, the mysterious viruses had intrigued scientists. When they couldn't identify visible bacteria under optical microscopes in a number of contagious diseases such as small pox, chicken pox and rabies, they suspected a smaller, invisible microbe. Pasteur, in 1884, unable to find the bacteria causing rabies, declared it must be "a microorganism infinitesimally small."

Iwanowski in 1892 was the first to identify as the cause of tobacco leaf disease, an organism so small it passed through a porcelain filter fine enough to keep back ordinary bacteria. Although he never saw the microorganism, it came to be called the tobacco mosaic *virus*. From this beginning, scientists made rather slow progress in studying viruses and recognized effects of viruses long before actually seeing the "infinitesimally small" microorganisms themselves.

A myxomatous tumor of rabbits, studied by Sanarelli of Uruguay in 1898, was the first contagious disease and the first cancer recognized to be transmissible by a microscopically invisible agent. The organism caused benign fibromas in wild rabbits but fatal myxomas in domestic rabbits.

In 1907 a German investigator, Marek, described a disease of fowls in which rapidly proliferating lymphoid cells infiltrated nerves, producing tumors and paralysis. Since the disease was obviously a cancer, yet highly infectious for chickens, he assumed it to be due to a virus. The following year in Copenhagen, Ellermann and Bang took blood from a chicken with leukemia, filtered it of all cells, and injected the remaining fluid into a healthy chicken, which later developed leukemia.

In 1911 Peyton Rous in New York's Rockerfeller Institute transmitted a chicken sarcoma to healthy fowls with a cell-free filtrate of the tumor. Twenty years later, in 1932, at the Rockerfeller Institute in Princeton, New Jersey, Richard Shope transmitted a rabbit fibroma by cell-free filtrates. In 1936, John Bittner demonstrated that mouse breast cancer could be passed from the mother to a nursing female mouse that later also developed breast cancer.

Baldwin Lucke in Philadelphia suggested a viral cause for a kidney cancer found in frogs in 1938. By injecting cell-free filtrate obtained from leukemic mice, Ludwik Gross in 1951 induced leukemia in newborn mice.

All these instances of cancer being transmitted from one animal to another implicated an infectious virus. Stewart and Eddy at the National Institutes of Health in 1957 found they could propagate a parotid tumor virus in tissue culture. They called it a "polyoma virus," since it could induce a variety of tumors not only in mice, but also in rats and hamsters.

In 1935 Ledingham and Gye demonstrated tiny particles by high speed centrifugation of a filtrate from the Rous sarcoma. They believed these 70-millimicron-sized particles to be the Rous sarcoma virus (a millimicron is one-millionth of a millimeter).

When the electron microscope was introduced about 1945, it offered for the first time the possibility of actually seeing viruses. As early as 1946, Claude, Porter and Pickels examined Rous cells under the electron microscope and reported dense particles, about 75 millimicrons in size, scattered in the cytoplasm of some of the cells. Anthony Epstein in 1956 correlated morphological and biological aspects of the Rous virus, definitely identifying Rous virus particles of 70 millimicron size.

Because for years scientists had identified a variety of infective cancer viruses in animals, many virologists engaged in this type of investigation, were now eager to be the first to find a virus causing a human cancer. The African lymphoma, with its peculiar geographic pattern, had all the characteristics of a human tumor caused by a biologic agent, most likely a virus. This is why it was becoming the focus of intensive international study.

*****

Burkitt's friend, Dr. Bill Davis, the director of the Uganda Colonial Medical Services who had allowed him time for his safari, indicated one day that he would like to have a chat, so Olive invited him to lunch at their home. It proved to be an unforgettable occasion. Both Denis and Olive knew that something important was on Davis's mind as he sat at their table, for he had some difficulty in carrying on his usually uninhibited conversation.

At last, after the dessert had been savored and Yusufu had taken the dishes from the table, Davis cleared his throat. "Denis," he began, "you of course know about Uganda's upcoming independence. You must realize that the new government will want to employ its own African physicians, whose salaries are less than those of ex-patriot doctors. Unfortunately, Denis, you've been working yourself out of a job, training capable African surgeons all these years."

This was a shock, and quite unexpected. Denis hardly knew what to say. After a long pause, he asked, "What suggestion do you have for me?"

"It might be prudent," the director advised, "if you'd consider resigning from your position at the hospital within a few months."

"Under the circumstances," Denis said, standing up from the table, "I suppose that's the only thing I can do. Thanks for the warning." But to himself he was thinking, *What am I to do? At age 51, there's little chance I could get a surgical appointment in England with my too broad, nonspecialized surgical experience. And besides, what will come of all my research? I've only just begun to get to the bottom of the lymphoma puzzle!*

That evening, after he and Olive had discussed the situation and prayed about it, Denis wrote in his diary for June 22, 1962: "Not really worried. The Lord will open the way." It took faith for him to write those words, little dreaming just how wonderfully the way would be opened before him. He decided not to resign, but just to wait.

In less than two weeks, Ian McAdam approached him with a suggestion. "You ought to consider going full-time into geographical medicine. It's a relatively new area of medical research. That's what you've already been doing with the African lymphoma, Denis. Your studies are nothing less than geographical medicine in the purest sense."

Burkitt looked hopefully at his friend. "It's true, I've been doing this type of medical practice in my spare time. But," he questioned, "who would ever hire me to do this kind of research on a full-time basis?"

"I've an idea," Ian encouraged him, "and will try to pursue something for you. I don't want the lymphoma project coming to nothing any more than you do. I believe I'm the one to work on this problem until it's solved." On this promising note, the friends parted.

Once more Denis and Olive discussed at length his professional future. "Ian has suggested that I forget my surgical practice and go into geographical medicine, which is what I've been doing in the lymphoma research already. He said he'd look into the possibility for me. What do you think?"

"We've been praying something would open up," Olive said, "and maybe this is what God has in mind for you. I've just been reading First Samuel, the tenth chapter, and couldn't but notice how after Samuel anointed Saul to be king, he gave him specific instructions to follow. As Saul followed the prophet's step-by-step commands, everything happened just as Samuel said it would. I believe the Lord will similarly open the way for you, Denis, if you just follow His leading."

Denis gave her a hug, saying how much he appreciated the loving, loyal wife the Lord had given him. "You always encourage me when I most need it ."

That night he wrote in his diary: "Feeling at peace over Ian's suggestion."

Early in July, Denis went down to the British virus laboratory in Entebbe to observe their investigations on the tumor. There had been excitement in the laboratory months before, when they'd found a Reo Type 3 virus in lymphoma tissue. Following this discovery, they had injected rabbits with large doses of the recovered Reo Type 3 virus. Only recently, one of the rabbits had developed a lump, which they had removed and taken to Dr. Wright in Kampala for tissue diagnosis. At first, Dr. Wright thought it might actually be the lymphoma, but after making additional preparations of the tissue, he diagnosed a myeloma, a plasma cell tumor. With considerably more study, the team reluctantly decided that the Reo Type 3 virus was merely associated as a "passenger" in the tumor and not as the causative agent.

*****

A much-needed, modern, six-storied Mulago Hospital was now nearing completion in Kampala. This facility would be more representative, as streams of visitors continued to inquire about Burkitt's work on the African lymphoma. Denis had recently enjoyed two hours with Colonel Blomberg, director from the Armed Forces Institute of Pathology, in Washington, D.C.

In August, the presidents of both the Edinburgh and the English Colleges of Surgeons, Sir John Bruce and Sir Arthur Porritt, visited simultaneously. Ian, wishing to impress these eminent physicians, properly, suggested to his surgical staff, "In the lecture theater, present some of our unusual patients for them, the likes of which they'll be unlikely to see in the United Kingdom."

With these orders, surgeon Odonga brought in a man covered with bandages and announced, "Here is a type of trauma with which you are probably unacquainted—severe hippopotamus bites." He proceeded to discuss the frequency and seriousness of such cases.

Dr. Shepard next presented a man with an enormous groin hernia. He grossly exaggerated, saying with a smile, "At Mulago Hospital, we have three categories for hernias: those not reaching the knee, those reaching below the knee and those touching the floor!"

Finally, Denis brought in four children, each with four-jaw involvement of the lymphoma—sixteen tumors in the four children. At that time, only seventeen tumors of this kind had been reported in world medical literature. In presenting the cases, Denis said, "Here stand the near-equivalent of all the jaw lymphoma patients reported in the world!" Needless to say, the British surgeons were first amused, then impressed.

*****

Burkitt had received an all-expense-paid invitation to lecture at the famous cancer research center, the Sloane-Kettering Institute in New York City. Now, in August, a request came to lecture and attend a conference on viruses and cancer at the M.D. Anderson Hospital in Houston, Texas. Since both invitations were scheduled for the following February, he figured it would be possible to accept both.

Before these appointments, however, he was to attend the biannual meeting of the South African Association of Surgeons. The Association notified Denis that as the opening guest speaker for this formal occasion, he should wear a dinner jacket and black tie. Years before, he had acquired a jacket from one uncle and trousers from another to make up a dinner suit, but this outfit seemed hardly appropriate. Where could he find a formal dinner suit in tropical, unsophisticated Kampala? Olive searched in all the stores, and then came upon an ad for a used coat-and-trouser-dinner outfit in the local paper. Denis felt fortunate, indeed, when this secondhand "proper" suit fit perfectly, especially as he acquired it for a very reasonable price.

In September, he flew to Johannesburg for the meeting. His address, given at a formal dinner in the evening, preceded the scientific sessions. It was at the formal dinner that he had to appear in the dinner jacket and black tie. To his relief, for this was his first talk on the subject before a large international audience, the surgeons received his lecture on the African lymphoma well.

When he returned to Kampala, Ian McAdam had good news for him. Ian reported that he had corresponded with Sir Harold Himsworth, director of the British Medical Research Council in London. Himsworth had previously met Burkitt on a visit to Kampala and had arranged for a sizable, supporting, research grant. McAdam had written him to say that Burkitt would soon be available and suggested that he take him on his staff as a full-time research worker before someone else "lapped him up."

Denis laughed at the "blarney" Ian had dished out.

"Of course Himsworth wanted you," McAdam exulted, "and here's the best news of all. You're to stay right here in Kampala. You'll have the same office, the same secretary, the same old friends! But now, instead of doing routine surgery, you'll be free to do epidemiology full time." Ian slapped Denis on the shoulder. "Could anything be better?"

"How can I thank you, Ian? You've certainly encouraged me!" Denis turned away, heading home to tell Olive the great news.

She accepted the word as God's will. Denis realized that Olive might personally have preferred to return to England. In just a week, Cassy would again be flying to England for school. Judy had been away for two years, attending a school in the Kenya highlands. Their biggest sacrifice living in Kampala, was that each of their daughters, after the age of twelve, had to leave home for her education. Rachel, however, was still at home, but would have to go to boarding school in another year.

*****

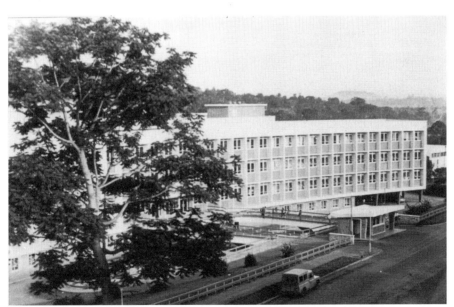

The beautiful new Mulago Hospital, 1962.

Uganda was to be the second East African territory, after Tanzania, to gain independence from Britain. Bill Davis appointed Denis as the official physician for the Duke and Duchess of Kent, who were representing Queen Elizabeth II on a state visit to celebrate Ugandan independence. On October 7, he and Olive went to Entebbe to meet the royal couple, and from then on, accompanied them throughout their ten-day visit, including their excursions to the game parks. The evening after the royal couple's arrival, October 8, 1962, the Burkitts had special seats near the Duke and Duchess who, in the name of the Queen, relinquished British rule to the new Uganda government. Denis and Olive watched at midnight the poignant moment when the Union Jack was slowly lowered and the new Uganda flag raised, signifying the transfer of power, from Britain to Uganda, under the new leadership of Milton Obote.

During the same visit, the Duchess on October 16 officially opened the sparkling new Mulago Hospital. In her dedicatory speech she mentioned the lymphoma studies which were attracting scientists from around the world to the institution. This was not to be the last time the Burkitts would meet the Duchess of Kent. The next time, over twenty years in the future, she would honor Denis himself.

Of all the many contacts Denis made during these exciting years in Kampala, perhaps the most meaningful in terms of a close, lasting friendship was with Ralph and Ruth Blocksma. The Blocksma's initial visit to Uganda came in early November. Denis had just emerged from his office when he met a stranger coming down the hall. Ever the friendly welcomer, he stretched out his hand, saying, "Denis Burkitt."

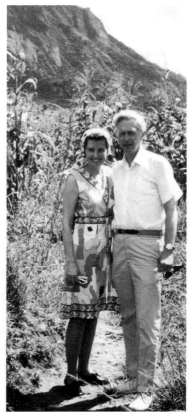

Blocksma shook his hand and introduced himself as a plastic surgeon from Grand Rapids, Michigan. Hesitating a bit and smiling, he added, "I've just met one of your fellow doctors. Your friend said, with humor, of course, 'You should meet the "strange" man down the hall who's just finished a 10,000 mile safari. He'll talk your head off about his project!' That kind of introduction has made me curious."

Burkitt laughed enthusiastically and said, "If you have a few minutes, I'd love to show you our medical mystery." Denis took the visiting surgeon by the arm and steered him into his office, where the most obvious attraction was the button-festooned map of Africa on the wall.

As Burkitt excitedly reviewed information on the childhood tumor, he added, "Since you're a surgeon, you can appreciate how frus-

Ralph and Ruth Blocksma.

126

trating it has been dealing with a cancer which can't be excised. Recently, however, we've found these tumors are responsive to Methotrexate or Endoxan injections. Chemotherapy is giving real hope to these children."

As their conversation, which had become quite lengthy, continued, Denis learned that the Blocksmas had formerly been medical missionaries in Pakistan. Soon after the partition of Pakistan from India, they had started a mission hospital there, sponsored by the United Reform Church. Unfortunately, Ruth had developed severe complications of amebiasis accompanying a pregnancy, and because of other health hazards to the children, the mission board wouldn't allow them to return following their home leave. They were greatly disappointed, but Ralph conceived the idea of "tithing his time" (five or six weeks a year) to missions, even writing an article on the subject for the *Christian Medical Society Journal*.

After their return to the States, Ralph had resumed his specialty practice of plastic surgery at the Butterworth Hospital in Grand Rapids. Before long, he developed a teaching program and trained plastic surgeons who would afterward be working all over the world. Because of his earlier exposure to overseas medical needs, he enjoyed serving and lecturing abroad whenever the opportunity arose, as he "tithed his time." His reason for presently being in Kampala was that he'd been invited to give a series of lectures at Makerere Medical School.

Burkitt seized his opportunity and told Ralph of the weekly Bible studies in his home. He invited Ralph to give the current week's study, knowing he would receive an affirmative reply. This was the beginning of an enduring friendship. Before leaving Kampala, the Blocksmas extracted a promise from the Burkitts to visit them in Grand Rapids, should they ever come to the States.

*****

Before the end of the year, Makerere appointed Dr. Michael Hutt as the new professor of pathology at the medical school. As Burkitt became acquainted with Dr. Hutt, he learned that he was also a committed Christian. While a senior lecturer and consultant at St. Thomas's Medical School in London, Hutt and his wife had begun entertaining African physicians who attended their church. These doctors, in turn, encouraged him to consider a teaching career in Africa.

Hutt had read Denis's *Cancer* article with considerable interest. So, a few months later in 1961, when he turned to the back pages of the *British Medical Journal* and saw a notice requesting applications for the Professorship of Pathology at Makerere, he was immediately attracted. After discussing with his wife the possibility of an assignment in Africa, he applied and was appointed to the post.

As Hutt was considering the vastness of his scientific field soon after his arrival in Kampala, and wondering where he should concentrate, the Professor of Pediatrics,

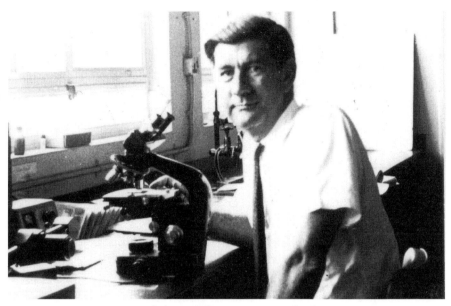

New pathology professor, Doctor Michael Hutt.

Dick Jelliffe, gave him excellent advice. "Don't paint miniatures. Paint on a wide scale." It wasn't long before Michael Hutt had a special interest in geographical pathology, realizing its importance in studying various diseases.

Not unexpectedly, he and Burkitt spent considerable time together discussing the potential contributions the African lymphoma could have to an understanding not only of the tumor itself, but of cancer in general. It would be the geographical limitations of the disease, he was certain, that would help uncover the cause of the disease. Hutt assured Denis he would work closely with him on the lymphoma project.

"I'd like to start a new plan before long," Hutt told Burkitt, "and that is to offer free diagnostic pathology services to all mission hospitals in Uganda, as well as to the government hospitals. This will encourage biopsy diagnoses on all lymphoma cases and benefit your research."

"That's an excellent idea," Denis agreed. "There are too many accessible lesions never confirmed by biopsy diagnosis, simply because of the cost." From then on, the Mulago Hospital supplied free for the asking, boxes containing formalin-filled biopsy bottles. The response from hospitals throughout the country was gratifying to the new Chief of Pathology.

*****

Denis had been preparing three papers for presentation at a conference in early 1963 on "Tumors of the Lympho-Reticular System in Africa." The scheduled conference was to be held at Dakar, Senegal, in West Africa. He and two other doctors from Makerere had arranged their flight across Africa with the Flying Doctors. However, the current African political situation wouldn't permit the South African delegates to go to a medical conference in Senegal. In fact, at the time, for political reasons, there was no place on the African continent open to every delegate. Thus the location of the conference was changed to Paris. Its date in February, dovetailed perfectly with Denis's plans for his first trip to the United States in the same month.

After thirteen-year-old Cassy left for England the previous fall, Denis tried to write her faithfully, knowing her longings for her family. From Paris on February 15 he wrote:

> Dear Cass:
>
> Thank you so much for your letter addressed to me here.
>
> Paris is a lovely city, but everything is terribly expensive. I had an 18/- lunch yesterday and had to buy a piece of chocolate after it to satisfy my hunger. The excellent lunch at the Uganda Club costs 5/-.
>
> I am so glad that Mummy has Aunt Lucy with her while I am away. I am naturally looking forward very much to seeing you on Saturday fortnight.
>
> Strange to say an East African paper called the *Register* came out with my photograph on the front page and an article on the tumor. I have brought you a copy for fun. On Saturday, I fly to America. My days are spent in conference, so I haven't seen much of Paris.
>
> God bless, and very dear love from your
>
> > Daddy

The Paris meeting was a momentous occasion for Denis, as it was almost entirely devoted to discussion of the African childhood tumor. Even though eminent pathologists from around the world recognized it as a newly described lymphoma, they couldn't agree on its exact classification. More intensive studies of the tumor cells themselves would be necessary, employing many emerging new research techniques in order to designate the exact type of primitive lymphocyte composing it.

However, a recognized name needed to be appended to the cancer so that when referring to it in scientific circles, all would understand the nomenclature. Already in most of Africa the cancer was referred to as "Burkitt's tumor," in view of his initial description and research on it. So, because they were unable to agree on the true nature of the lymphoma, it was decided at this conference to call it officially "Burkitt's tumor." (Somewhat later, the name was changed to "Burkitt's lymphoma," a term better specifying its cancerous nature).

It was a heady honor for Denis, to see his name used in medical literature throughout the world. He had a laugh, however, several months later to find that his daughter Judy, long before the conference, had loyally written in her diary, "They ought to call it *Burkitt's Tumor.*"

From Paris, Denis flew on February 16 to New York. Because there were several days before his appointment at the M.D. Anderson Hospital, he chose to travel to Houston by train in order to see as much of the countryside as possible. But, on reaching New Orleans, he was given a telegram requesting that he fly immediately to Dallas for consultation on a possible Burkitt's lymphoma patient there. The additional expense for his detoured flight to Dallas would be reimbursed. It was immensely exciting to examine a possible case outside tropical Africa! What would be the geographical and viral implications now?

Denis got off the train, boarded a plane, and was shortly examining the patient and discussing the case in Dallas. The patient *did have* Burkitt's lymphoma, but he was at a loss to explain why a person in Texas, so far removed from the tropics, should have it! Here was another piece in the puzzle. Would they ever be able to put everything together?

In Houston, Denis was aghast at the grandeur of the Hilton Hotel. He had never seen, let alone actually enjoyed, such luxury. To be able to take a bath with water more than covering the legs seemed almost a sin! He made careful note of every spectacular feature to relate to Olive. How he wished she might have been there to enjoy it with him.

The whole conference was on viruses and nucleic acids, far over his head, as he later confessed. His was nearly the last talk and he was afraid it was too "down to earth" after all the erudite chemistry presentations. But his dramatic pictures of Africa and its unfortunate children bearing the lymphoma, accompanied by explanations in his clear Irish brogue interspersed occasionally with humor, won the audience, who gave him a standing ovation. They

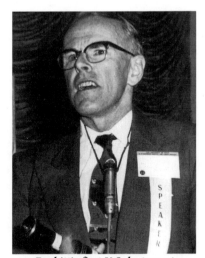

Burkitt's first U.S. lecture at Houston's M.D. Anderson Hospital.

made him an honorary citizen of the state of Texas, so designated with a card signed by Governor Connally.

His lecture at the Sloane-Kettering Institute in New York was almost an anticlimax after the Texas reception. He was indebted to this institute for contributing funds toward his fact-finding safari and specifically to its Joe Burchenal, who had started the lifesaving chemotherapy for the stricken lymphoma children at Mulago. Denis expressed his thanks profusely. With transparencies taken on safari, he pictured the fruits of their support and demonstrated dramatic results of chemotherapy by before-and-after photos of characteristic tumor cases.

His visit to the institute proved a rare opportunity for him to meet various eminent scientists who were working on the leukemia-lymphoma problem, including Dr. Gross, who had transmitted mouse leukemia into newborn mice fifteen years earlier.

Flying to England, he looked forward to a brief visit with Cassy at the Westonbirt School in Tetbury. That evening, after their visit, he wrote Cassy a note:

My dear Cass:

I am sitting in my rather cold attic bedroom after my day with you.

What a joy it was being able to meet like that. We both talked rather superficially trying to be cheerful, and yet I know we longed for a deeper contact. The moment of separation revealed this and it was then I realized how much my Cass meant to me. I think for the first time in saying goodbye to you or Judy, I cried. I couldn't stop, and I know you cried too. I knew how deep the bonds that held us together and I wiped many tears from my face on the journey back to Farnham Common.

You will be very especially in my prayers as you try to stand for all that is good and best. I shall look forward with longing to gathering you up from the school again in July.

I needn't write more. You know how much I loved seeing you.

Very very dear love, your

Daddy

In London he visited briefly with Tony Epstein and others interested in his research, before returning to Uganda and Olive.

*****

Judy, home from her school in the African highlands for the Easter holiday, was as anxious as ever to help her father with his maps, charts or whatever she was capable of doing for him. As he went through the mass of mail which had collected on his desk during his absence, he opened a letter from New Guinea. Several weeks earlier, he had sent a questionnaire to mission hospitals in other tropical countries, hoping possibly to learn the worldwide extent of the tumor. As he read the letter, his excitement grew. It advised him that the lymphoma was common in New Guinea, being recognized now for the first time from his descriptions.

Another report added one more puzzling piece to the ever-more-complex lymphoma riddle. A rather high incidence of **adult cases** of the tumor was now being reported in Uganda among recent immigrants from the highlands of Burundi and Rwanda. Why should these persons coming from areas where the tumor didn't exist, acquire the cancer in Uganda? And why adults? It was something new. This development was disturbing, for the reason was not yet apparent.

It's time, thought Denis, *for all our bits of information to come together and make sense!*

11

FINDING THE VIRUS CONNECTION

In July 1963 there was no magical Laragh to visit in Ireland, so the Burkitts spent the first few weeks of their home-leave shifting uneasily between a rented cottage in West Ireland and the home of relatives near Cork. Denis enjoyed briefly reliving his childhood by showing Olive and the girls his Grandfather Thomas Burkitt's former manse near Galway, where he and Robin had played years before.

Since both Denis and Olive had been invited by the Sloane-Kettering Institute for an expense-paid, return trip by ship to New York, they said goodbye at the end of September to Cassy and Rachel, now enrolled in English schools. In spite of crossing the Atlantic in a luxurious cabin with wonderful food, Olive did not enjoy the voyage, for she was seasick most of the time. However, as their ship entered the New York harbor, they both experienced the thrill of millions before them in viewing the Statue of Liberty.

Denis's correspondence with scientists across the United States had resulted in so many invitations to lecture that he'd planned a mammoth American "safari." Once more he met his friend Joe Burchenal when he delivered his scheduled lecture at the Sloane-Kettering Institute in New York. From there, he and Olive traveled by bus to Washington D.C., where, friends met, lodged, and toured them. Burkitt lectured at the prestigious Armed Forces Institute of Pathology at the invitation of its director Colonel Blomberg, whom he had met in Kampala.

Lectures followed in Buffalo, Toronto, Kingston and London, Ontario, as well as in Grand Rapids, Michigan, where they enjoyed the hospitality of their new friends, the Blocksmas.

Since Ralph Blocksma had been the first president of the Medical Assistance Program (M.A.P.), an organization collecting and distributing drugs and medical supplies free to medical missionaries throughout the world, he suggested that Burkitt really should meet Ray Knighton, its director. Ralph visualized how this organization could greatly benefit Burkitt's research program and arranged for Denis and Olive to stay with Knighton and his wife in Chicago. Through Knighton, Denis learned of the worldwide work of this philanthropic foundation.

But the constant strain of travel and meeting new people was fatiguing for Olive, who began feeling tired and ill. The previous few months had given her no respite as she had packed all their household belongings ready to move into a different house on their return to Uganda, in addition to packing for their home leave. They had been unsettled for weeks, visiting relatives in Ireland and England. Finally, it had fallen her responsibility to locate schools in England for Cassy and Rachel as well as arrange for Judy's return for continued schooling in Kenya. Now the rigorous American trip was upon her.

Olive in no way wanted to interfere with the opportunities that were opening for Denis. However, on the train between Chicago and San Francisco, she began feeling wretched. What were they to do? Denis still had extensive commitments, not only in the United States but also in Canada. He decided to phone the Blocksmas for their counsel.

"Put Olive on the train. We'll meet her in Chicago and take care of her like a mother and father until you come back," was their solution. The Blocksma's thoughtful invitation made even more firm the growing bond between the two families.

In San Francisco, Denis lectured to several hundred of the 5,000 attendants at the American Surgical Society meeting, an exhilarating experience, for he had never before spoken to a crowd of more than 200. Denis had two objectives on this North American tour: not only to fulfill speaking appointments for scientific audiences, but also to make appearances at Christian Medical Society gatherings.

By Greyhound bus, he traveled to Portland and Vancouver, keeping engagements in these cities. Then, catching a train, he traveled across Canada, stopping for lectures in Saskatchewan, Edmonton, and Winnipeg. On arriving back in Toronto, he phoned Olive at the Blocksmas' and arranged to meet her at the airport in Pittsburgh. Although they were still scheduled to return to England by ship, he canceled their reservations and purchased plane tickets instead, as Olive was still not well.

On their return to England in November, they rented a house in Nettlebed, near Oxford. This was to be Denis's and Olive's darkest hour, for he was due to return in about a month to his exciting work in Uganda. But Olive was depressed, even as she had been after Rachel's birth. Several times a day, Denis and Olive went for long walks, but her improvement was slow.

After much discussion and prayer, their final plan was for Olive to stay in England over Christmas so that she could be with the girls during the holidays. Denis, in the meantime, would return alone to Uganda to carry on his work. Denis often silently prayed, *Lord, what should I do? How can I abandon my dear wife when she needs me so, and yet You've given me a work in Africa. What should I really do?* Their December parting was harder than any they had heretofore experienced.

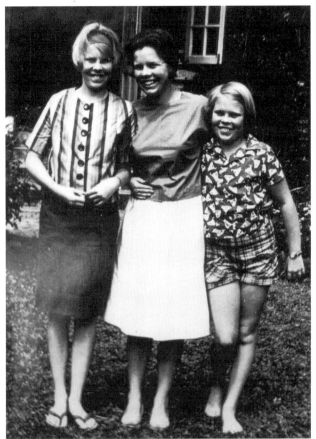

Left to right: Cassy, Judy and Rachel enjoy vacation at home in Kampala.

Back in Uganda alone at the beginning of 1964, one of Denis's first jobs was to move all the household goods Olive had packed from the Mulago Hill house where they had lived for the past fifteen years to another house a mile away. Since he was no longer on the surgical service and was not needed near the hospital, he vacated his longtime house for a successor.

With his new responsibilities in geographical medical research facing him, he had to formulate a plan of what to do next. As he looked over his lymphoma maps, he thought, *Here is the distribution of the cancer we've found from our safaris. We all think there must be some virus that's responsible for the tumor. Could it be that an insect vector injects the virus directly into the blood stream of a child, causing the tumor?* This was hardly a new thought to Denis. The idea had haunted him for years.

He took out several maps of disease distribution and studied them closely. *The only places in the world where malaria is hyper-endemic are in tropical parts of Africa, New Guinea, Malaysia, and parts of the Amazon basin. I've written to doctors in all these areas and have already heard that the lymphoma is present in New Guinea.*

Now, there are only two places in the whole of tropical Africa with a year-round high temperature and rainfall where the tumor doesn't occur. These are the Islands of Zanzibar on the east coast of Tanzania and Leopoldville (Kinshasa) in Zaire. Looking closely at malaria control charts, he noticed, *Zanzibar and Kinshasa are the only parts of tropical Africa where malaria has been successfully eradicated. The eradication of malaria must be due to regular mosquito spraying in these places.*

He now had figures to calculate the incidence of lymphoma per 100,000 population in various districts. Denis recalled that there had been a recent survey of malaria density in Uganda. *Look at that!* he exclaimed aloud. *In every district where malaria is intensive, there are great numbers of the tumor, and vice versa. There seems to be a **direct relationship between the incidence of intense malaria infection and the lymphoma**. Why should that be?* It now became obvious to Denis, that on their 10,000 mile safari, they had actually mapped areas of high-malaria-density.

On February 6, he received a discouraging letter from Olive. She still wasn't well, and although the holidays had long since passed, she still didn't feel able to make the trip to Uganda. This made him apprehensive. In his Bible study that evening he found comfort in Psalm 86:16: "O turn unto me, and have mercy upon me; give thy strength unto thy servant…"

However, on the 8th, he received a phone call from London. Olive's physician asked him to fly home to be with her. Within a couple of days he was on a plane, flying to Olive, his mind in a whirl. All he could think of was the verse in Psalm 30:5: "Weeping may endure for a night, but joy cometh in the morning."

A week after arriving back in England, he wrote in his diary: "Future dark, but opening a little." They enjoyed long walks, and gradually she began to improve. Some of the time he spent writing on his next medical paper. Also, he was asked to appear on a television program discussing viruses.

On February 28, his birthday, he made this entry: "Olive longs for a home in England soon. My work makes it yet impossible. I cry to God for peace and guidance. A very difficult time." March 5, he wrote: "Beginning work on lymphoma book with Dennis Wright. We made a trip to see the girls at school." March 18: "Olive feeling better." He made plans to return to Uganda on the 21st, and wrote in his diary on March 20: "Very difficult day. Both feeling tomorrow's parting so much. Oh God, give us all the strength and peace we need!" March 21: "Left Olive for the most difficult parting of our lives."

*****

On his return to Kampala, Dennis Wright met him with exciting news. "Did you see Tony Epstein in London?" he asked.

"Not recently, " Denis answered, his curiosity aroused. "Why do you ask?"

"Tony didn't know where you were, so he wrote me some *most interesting* news." Wright knew that Denis would want all the details as he continued, "In early December Tony received a biopsy sample from us which had been delayed en route from Mulago. It arrived late on a Friday afternoon, and when he examined the specimen, he found a cloudy fluid surrounding the tissue. Everyone in the lab wanted to go home for the weekend. One of the workers suggested that Tony trash the specimen, since it appeared to be contaminated with bacteria."

"Did he throw out the specimen?" Denis wanted to know.

"Fortunately, he didn't," continued Wright. "He decided to make a wet mount of the fluid for a quick examination under the microscope, and was surprised to find no bacteria. Instead, he saw clumps of what appeared to be viable tumor cells. So he decided to culture these cells that he found in the fluid suspension."

"Did the tumor cells grow in the culture?" Denis asked, standing on one leg and then the other, impatiently waiting for the *most interesting news.*

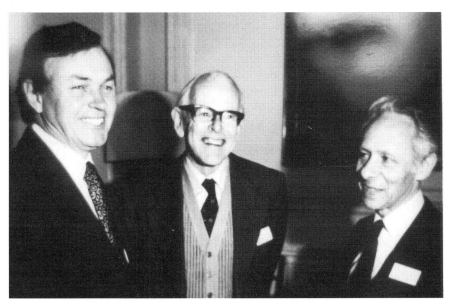

Burkitt (center) and Anthony Epstein (right). (Later Picture.)

"Tony wrote that it had taken seventy-five days to culture out sufficient material so he could make thin sections for electron microscopic examination. As he was looking at the first grid, he immediately found a cell with numerous virus particles." Wright paused to watch the expression on Denis's face. "Tony said he was so excited, he had turned off the microscope for fear the light might burn up the viruses. He took a walk around the block to cool his head a bit before returning to the lab. Then he gathered his co-workers around him, turned on the light, and they all saw that the virus particles were still there!"

Burkitt drew a deep breath. "Was he able to identify the type of virus?"

"He recognized the particles as having a typical herpes morphology, but he hasn't identified the specific type yet. He thinks it may be a new type of herpes virus. If this proves to be the viral agent we've been suspecting for a long time, he will have found the first human cancer-causing virus, and February 24, 1964, the date of his finding them, will be important in medical history!" Wright finished.

Burkitt was still cautious, even though greatly excited. "Let's hope his diligence has paid off. He's been working away on this for two years now. Of course, it will take time to determine if this virus is really the causative agent of the lymphoma or only a passenger like the Reo Type 3."

*****

In mid-April, Epstein returned to Kampala to check on the monkeys he had inoculated with tumor tissue two years previously. He found that two of the three monkeys had peculiar lumps in their arm and leg long-bones. Upon x-raying the bones of the affected monkeys, he found that both animals had multiple "green stick" fractures in the areas of tumor-like growth. The affected bones showed dark-red areas when biopsied. Microscopic study of the tissue revealed sheets of cells, which at first were thought to be tumor. However, when Dennis Wright reviewed the slides, he could not make that diagnosis.

A disappointed Tony Epstein had no sooner left Kampala than Ted Williams appeared at Burkitt's office door. Denis greeted him warmly, "Ted, it's been some time since I've seen you." Denis pulled a chair over for him to sit down. "The pathologists say you're sending in quite a few biopsies for confirmation on lymphoma cases."

Ted sat down and crossed his legs. "You know, Denis," he began, "you really inspired me on the safari. I've found that our West Nile district is a hotbed of lymphoma cases, so I've been careful to get pathological confirmation on each child. I can really thank Michael Hutt for instigating the new biopsy service. With this information, I've been plotting each case, noting the exact home location of the child on a map."

"That's great!" Denis approved. "Have you found anything new?"

"That's why I'm here," Ted said. "I've noticed during this last year that several lymphoma patients have lived in close proximity to each other, and I've wondered if you think there could be any significance to this."

Burkitt tapped his pen slowly on his desk before answering. "There just might be. I have an idea. Hutt and I are going up into your area in a few days. This will give us an opportunity to look over your records and map. We'd also like to see, first hand, the home areas of these cases." Denis rose and pushed back his chair from the desk. "We'll see you at Kuluva in a few days."

So, as a follow-up to Ted's request, Burkitt and Michael Hutt drove up to Kuluva by Land Rover and were shortly inspecting a designated locale where a small "epidemic" of lymphoma cases had occurred. They also scrutinized Ted's records and map.

"Ted, you're certainly to be complimented on your careful observations and record-keeping," Hutt said. Turning to Burkitt, he added, "I'm impressed that he's on to something. We don't ordinarily see cancer cases in clusters like this. It's acting more like a contagious disease—and we now have Epstein's virus as a possible causative agent. This definitely needs further investigation!"

"Why don't we alert the Virus Research group in Entebbe," Denis suggested, "and have them follow this up with Ted?"

Ted nodded his head. "Good idea. I'll be looking for someone from Entebbe, and will be ready to help in any way I can."

*****

May 5, 1964 was a high day for Denis, for that day he brought Olive, feeling quite well, home to Kampala. Many friends met her with gifts and a lovely luncheon. Denis had just completed plans for several safari expeditions and given advanced notice to the various hospitals he hoped to visit. From now on, he hoped Olive would accompany him, if she wished, on all his safaris. There was no need for her to stay home, for Cassy and Rachel were attending school in England and Judy, in the highlands of Kenya.

His cancer interest had now widened to include not only information about the Burkitt's Lymphoma, designated "BL," but also six other cancers with apparent geographical distribution. These were cancers of the liver, esophagus, stomach, penis, and two skin cancers, Kaposi's sarcoma and a cancer occurring in tropical ulcer scars.

Denis and Olive left on May 20 for the first of many enjoyable trips. This first one was to the south and west of Uganda. They visited every hospital en route, many of which Burkitt had never visited or heard from previously. No sooner did they return home than they left again, on June 19, for an even longer safari into Tanzania and Kenya, traveling two to three hundred miles per day. They took in the Islands of Zanzibar, where no BL had been reported, and noted that the mosquitoes had indeed been eradicated there. No malaria had been reported in this area for a number of years.

July and August were special months, as the girls were all home on vacation. Happily, a new government policy allowed two paid, round-trip air fares per child during each eighteen-month service tour. All three girls were excited over Denis's work, volunteering to help with various assignments in his office. That summer he started giving Judy her promised driving lessons on an ideal site, an abandoned airstrip.

On August 8, he made a note in his diary of something most unusual: "Today I saw the first **spontaneous recovery in BL**. This is well-documented, with original pictures and a biopsy. The child had no treatment whatsoever. What can account for it?"

In early September, the whole family was able to go on a two-week safari into Kenya, thus giving the girls a new appreciation of their father's field work. Of course, he combined the expedition with enjoyable sightseeing. The week after their return home, all the girls were off to school again.

Olive was proving most helpful, not only in keeping records, but also in keeping him company. They thoroughly enjoyed each trip, planned for at least two weeks of every month. Coming back after these expeditions, there were stacks of mail to go through. Many invitations to lecture were coming in: Edinburgh, Royal College of Surgeons in London, Ethiopia, World Health Organization in Geneva, the makers of Endoxan (the chemotherapeutic agent he was using to treat BL) in Germany. New doors were opening.

In spite of their extended trips and busy office routine, Denis was always working on two or more papers for publication. As for Olive, there was his record-keeping to occupy her, as well as entertaining a constant stream of visitors when they were at home.

Denis entered another significant note in his diary on October 14: "Two BL children, thought to be incurable in spite of chemotherapy, turned up tumor-free. One child with advanced tumor causing paraplegia (paralysis of the lower body and legs) two years ago, walked in today with no evidence of the disease! Methotrexate and Endoxan are certainly miracle-working drugs." On October 18, he wrote as a proud father: "Judy is head girl of her school in Kenya this year and has just been accepted at the Teacher Training College in Cambridge." It seemed hardly possible that his little Judy would be seventeen in another two months.

*****

As 1964 progressed, Burkitt received more news of Epstein's virus from time to time. Tony had at first considered having British virologists help him identify his virus. However, within forty-eight hours of first identifying the viral particles, he decided to send his cell cultures to Werner and Gertrude Henle, well-known virologists at the Children's Hospital and University of Pennsylvania School of Medicine in Philadelphia.

Before long the Henles proved that the Epstein-Barr virus, so named from the first report of the virus in a 1964 *Lancet* article co-authored by Epstein, Achong and Barr, was a new type of herpes virus. Their investigation of the virus led them to a search for antibodies to the virus in the sera of Burkitt lymphoma patients, Nigerian children who had been flown for treatment to the National Institutes of Health in Bethesda, Maryland. (The body manufactures specific antibodies on exposure to the protein antigen part of a virus, and these antibodies circulate in the bloodstream. Finding this antibody in the serum of an individual, indicates previous exposure to the virus).

The Henles set about finding antibodies to the Epstein-Barr ("EB") virus by using an "indirect immunofluorescence test." The cultured lymphoblast cells containing the EB virus particles were first fixed to a glass slide. The blood serum from a Nigerian child, containing the suspected antibody, was next applied to the slide. If the antibody were present, it should attach to the specific protein antigen on the virus particles in the BL lymphoblasts. The next step was to wash the cells on the slide and add a nonspecific human antibody attached to a fluorescent dye. After the slide was incubated, the antibody-antigen reaction could be visualized and identified by its fluorescence under an ultraviolet microscope.

Using this indirect immunofluorescence test, the Henles tried antibodies of every known herpes virus type and found no fluorescence except with the serum from the Nigerian children with BL. Thus they confirmed that the **Epstein-Barr virus was a previously unrecognized herpes-type virus.**

To discover whether the Epstein-Barr virus ("EBV") was a causative factor in Burkitt's lymphoma, they had to answer certain questions.

> (1). Are antibodies to EBV present in all BL patients as they
> were in the Nigerian BL patients?

> (2). Are EBV antibodies found in persons with other diseases
> or in healthy persons?

> (3). If so, do patients with BL have a higher titer (concentra-
> tion) of the antibody than healthy people do?

Testing to see whether healthy people and those with other diseases also had the antibody, was the next step. They were more than surprised to discover that **a**

high percentage of all the healthy Americans they tested had the antibody to the EB virus! Could the EBV be a ubiquitous virus?

Then they learned the answer to the third question. **The Nigerian children whose sera they had been using had a titer of EBV antibody about ten times higher than healthy American children with the antibody.** After obtaining negative results using an additional wide range of virus-identification procedures, they determined that the Epstein-Barr virus was not a previously-known virus. However, under the electron microscope, the virus was quite similar to that found in the Lucke frog carcinoma. Also, the EBV had an antigen similar to that of a known animal tumor virus.

$$*****$$

In May 1964 Dennis Wright spent time in England pursuing the idea that if the EB virus was ubiquitous in the United States and Britain, there should be cases of Burkitt's lymphoma in English children. He went through twenty years' of records in a limited district of England, uncovering in this small study, nine cases of BL, formerly unrecognized. Gradually, cases of the lymphoma were being reported from other countries as well: India, Thailand, Hong Kong, Singapore, Malaysia, New Guinea, Australia, France, Norway, Finland and the United States. Burkitt now recalled the case of BL he'd seen in Dallas Texas several years earlier on his first trip to the United States.

With so many scientists currently interested in solving the lymphoma puzzle, Denis became even more excited when considering the far-reaching distribution and implications of his "humble" discovery, as he termed it. Was the EB virus actually a factor in *causing* the lymphoma, and if so, why did 85% of healthy people have antibodies to it? If most healthy people harbor the virus, what triggers it to cause cancer?

$$*****$$

To Burkitt, the fact that he was now widely in demand as a lecturer seemed incredible. Yet here was another invitation for May 1965, an important one-day conference in Washington D.C. at the National Institutes of Health. Again, the Medical Research Council gladly consented to his going. Both he and Dennis Wright attended the session. In June he was called to lecture in London. His trips to England always gave him the opportunity to take Cassy and Rachel out of school for a visit. When in Africa, he and Olive continued to go on lengthy safaris, and when not traveling, he was busy writing papers. During the summer, when all three girls were home, they were included on the trips, and, when in Kampala, they, as well as Olive, helped in his office.

More and more frequently Denis found that he was making notes in his diary regarding cured BL children. On May 9, 1965, he wrote: "Two symptom-free children returned." On May 23, he noted: "Namusisi I remembered well. This little girl was treated in 1960 and today is well." On September 25 he wrote: "Today I saw the first patient we ever completely cured (five years). He is fine. Lives ninety miles away."

In October, Denis and Olive made a safari into the north and east of Uganda, visiting Lira, their first station of nearly twenty years before. Imagine their surprise to find that their old house was now a seasonal residence of the new Prime Minister, Milton Obote.

And so their twenty-year Ugandan sojourn was soon to end. Their next home visit in 1966 would become a permanent move to England, where Denis was scheduled to continue his work with the Medical Research Council in London. Had the African experience been rewarding? Beyond anything Denis might have dreamed. Was it busy? Olive could affirm that! There seemed never to be a pause in their perpetual activity. Would this move to England prove the end of Burkitt's research possibilities? Hardly! He had opened a cornucopia of medical secrets just waiting to be properly arranged into a remarkable advance in cancer knowledge.

12

TAKING A NEW DIRECTION

During 1964 and 1965, Denis and Olive had made a total of eleven African safaris of 1,000 to 2,000 miles each, mostly over unpaved roads, visiting three or four hospitals a day. He had made three overseas lecture tours, speaking in seven countries.

It was during this time that he was awarded his first of many honors, the Harrison Prize from the Ear-Nose-Throat section of the Royal Society of Medicine. In early 1965, he had lectured on the African lymphoma at their meeting in London. This award he thought rather ironic, however, for it was his ENT appointment that he had so disliked during his surgery training in Preston many years before. In addition, it had been only in the early days at Mulago that he had ever done ENT surgery, simply because there was no one else to do it. Just imagine! His presentation before that society was considered the best of the year and the reason for the citation!

Before permanently leaving Uganda at the end of January 1966, he and Dr. Joe Burchenal, who had started the drug-treatment in Mulago, organized an International Cancer Conference on Burkitt's Lymphoma with emphasis on chemotherapy.

Scientists from all over the world came to Kampala. Weeks before the meeting, Denis made arrangements to bring from their homes all the "cured" children who could be found. Those coming from long distances were provided accommodation. The day before the conference began, he and Michael Hutt drove their cars into Entebbe to meet delegates arriving for the convention. Throughout the meetings, Olive prepared meals as they entertained various distinguished conferees in their home.

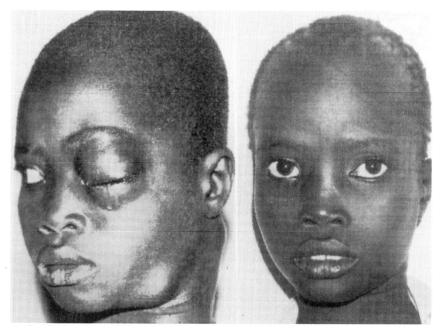

*Left: Child with Burkitt's lymphoma before treatment with chemotherapeutic drug.
Right: Same child after treatment.*

On January 5, the first day of the conference, Burkitt paraded, one by one, twenty-three normal-appearing children who had been successfully treated. He gave brief histories and exhibited photographs taken before treatment.

Next, Burkitt and Burchenal brought in several children with grotesquely swollen faces to demonstrate the appearance of the tumor before therapy. Following this initial presentation, they immediately started these children on Endoxan therapy. At the end of the conference, five days later, the same children again entered the conference hall. Their tumors had visibly regressed in this short time, a remarkable and impressive sight.

Among the notables in attendance were Professor Jean Barnard from Paris, Dr. Sarah Stewart of Sloane-Kettering, Dr. Neville Stanley from Australia, Dr. Bob Harris of the Imperial Cancer Research Fund, Sir Harold Himsworth from London's Medical Research Council, and Sir Alexander Haddow of the Chester Beatty Cancer Research Institute in London. Sir Haddow (not Alex Haddow, the entomologist) gave the closing address. In part, he said:

> I have been in the field of cancer research for nearly forty years; never in this time has the situation been more encouraging or more exciting. During this time I have attended hundreds of scientific meetings, yet with the utmost sincerity can I say that never have I attended a conference more fruitful or inspiring than this…As Dr. Burchenal had hoped, its [chemotherapeutic] effects

may be beneficial, not only for the treatment of children's cancer in Africa, but also for cancer therapy throughout the world...On the whole the conference has strengthened the case for the viral etiology of the Burkitt lymphoma; but equally right was Epstein when he described the viral evidence as possibly a "wild goose, but a goose that had to be chased." ...We are all, of course, extremely interested in the possibility that states of immune deficiency may lie behind the onset and course of malignant disease.

In closing, Dr. Haddow paid special tribute to Burkitt:

...an outstanding surgeon and, I would say, physician, an outstanding observer and researcher, but perhaps, beyond all else, what has most impressed us rests in his kindliness and in his humanity towards his patients, and we are all very proud of him.

*****

Denis, two weeks before leaving Kampala permanently, in spite of the pressures of the conference and preparations, as always took a few minutes to dash off a letter to Cassy in England:

Cass darling:

Now that our departure draws near we have invitations for every evening. We have provisionally refused some as we feel we must keep a day free for the department of Surgery. Our last Sunday we have tea with the Asian Christians, bless them.

Last week has been very busy. The conference on the so-called "Burkitt Tumour" went off exceedingly well. We had some 11 countries represented and all delegates seemed to enjoy and profit by the conference.

We had quite a lot of press cover from overseas more than locally. *Life* and *Time* magazines were interested and were sending long cables to their local representative so you might see me looking into a child's mouth in *Life* one day!

Mummy entertained some of the delegates to lunch and some to dinner in her always charming manner and had little poses of flowers sent to the ladies to wear at the minister's reception.... Next Sunday I speak at the Mulago Hospital service for the last time.

I have so many happy memories of speaking in the little chapel in the old Mulago.

Ranee is booked for Wednesday's plane. Her crate is very good and roomy...

Ladies of all races here are sad to think of Mummy going. I imagine she is one of the most universally loved ladies in Kampala. The wife of the High Commissioner is holding a special party for her. After tonight I don't think we will have a meal here until we go. How wonderful it has been to have such friends. We have hearts overflowing with thankfulness to the Lord for His mercies. People say what lovely daughters we have and I hope our family will be one that attracts people to come and see us and stay with us in England.

Very dear love,

Daddy

The following two weeks in Kampala were filled with final appointments of all kinds: Olive's last meeting with the young wives with whom she had been so active, a service with the Christian Medical Fellowship which Denis had helped found, his last talk at the Mulago chapel. Multiple farewell parties marked their imminent departure.

On January 25th they left from the Entebbe airport. To see them off at the plane was faithful Yusufu, only this time the broad gaps between his teeth were not noticeable, because he couldn't smile. The parting after his twenty years of friendship and faithfulness was equally hard for Denis and Olive. There, also in the crowd of well-wishers, stood the tall and slender Yudesi, the children's ayah since Rachel's birth. This committed Christian helper had always been trusted and loved.

As expected, Denis made the most of the trip. Their stop in Cairo was not only for viewing the various unrivaled antiquities, but also for meeting cancer specialists. They especially enjoyed visiting Jerusalem and environs where familiar Bible incidents had once transpired. He lectured there at the Weismann Institute. At length, after touring the impressive ruins of Athens, they reached London on the 14th of February.

Within a week, Denis noted in his diary the amusing difference between Kampala and riding with the crowds to his office on a commuter train to London. Under auspices of the Medical Research Council, he settled into his block of offices, where he had a fine secretary and before long a statistician, Paula Cook. She assisted him with his geographical studies on the seven-cancer project he was still pursuing in Africa.

The Research Council gave him a free hand to organize his studies and work as he wished. Needed expenses were paid for without question, as he had a reputation for extreme frugality. Already he began planning bigger East African undertakings. Just because he now had an office in London didn't mean he was abandoning his African investigations. Not at all! He hoped to continue making at least two, month-long African safaris a year.

Regarding the lymphoma project, Burkitt had been giving a lot of thought to the reason for the high predilection of the lymphoma for the jaws in young children. He and others suggested that the years for the maximal jaw tumor occurrence, about age eight, corresponded to the age of greatest dental development with disruption of the gingiva. This disruption might be giving opportunity for EB viruses to gain access to the tissues of the jaw.

Needless to say, it had never been Denis's nature to be idle. Since going to Africa in 1946, he had written by himself, or co-authored, forty-eight scientific papers

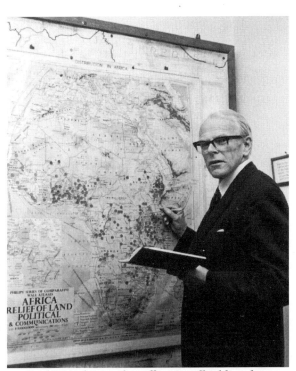

Burkitt, in his London office, is still adding data to his African map.

for publication. In more recent years, he had produced as many as eight or nine a year. During 1966 and 1967, he published twenty-five papers, eighteen of them in 1966, besides co-authoring a book with Burchenal on the treatment of Burkitt's tumor. During this two-year period he gave thirty lectures on several continents; attended seven international conferences, with lectures, and made three hectic African safaris. Little wonder on April 3, 1966, Olive's birthday, he noted in his diary: "This is the first time in seven years the whole family has been together for this occasion."

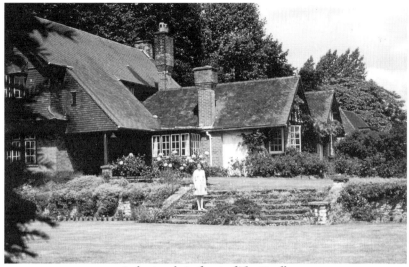

Judy stands in front of The Knoll.

Finding the ideal house in England was no small project. Denis estimated they must have looked at fifty houses, but finally, in late June, they found just the right one to meet their many needs and moved into it in mid-August. They were to spend the next twelve happy years at The Knoll, not infrequently having twelve to fifteen overnight guests. During a single year, they usually averaged over two hundred sleeping guests, not only many eminent scientists, but the especially enjoyable visits from young folks, friends of their girls.

It was after one weekend's entertainment of the girls' friends that Denis wrote a gentle reminder in a letter:

> Dearest Cass,
>
> I was so touched by your "Fathering Day" card on Sunday. I have brought it in and put it on my office desk. It is such loving spontaneous acts that count for so much in life and make the love of our daughters so very precious to us.
>
> With so much love,
>
> > Dad
>
> P.S. I left dear Mummy exceedingly weary this morning after an almost sleepless night, and yet she felt she must get up and get on with her work.

She is the one member of the family who has no let up. At weekends she is expected to get the breakfast and prepare the lunch and can never sleep in.

Please don't tell her I wrote this, but I know it grieved her that you should just dump your bed linen at the weekend expecting her to wash and iron it without even asking her. We all take it too much for granted that she is there to do the chores. It is just that you have vastly more spare time than she has. I know this was not selfishness but thoughtlessness, so I hope you won't mind my mentioning it. Last week she did your washing and ironing and I wonder if you even thanked her.

All this is meant to be *helpful* rather than critical.

Very dear love,

Daddy

*****

Burkitt's biggest tour at this time, came in October 1966. Beginning with a conference in Tokyo, he also took in Singapore, Hong Kong, Australia and New Guinea. In New Guinea, having previously heard of the presence of the lymphoma on the island, he and George Oettle from South Africa investigated the geographical distribution of the disease. They found it present, as expected, in coastal areas but not in the highlands. On the return trip to England, Denis passed through Bangkok, Karachi and Baghdad, as always, giving lectures.

Invariably, he had lunch with Tony Epstein two or three times a year, on which occasions he always learned the latest developments in the Epstein-Barr virus research. Late in 1967 he listened as Epstein told of a most remarkable incident which Denis could not consider mere serendipity. The incident happened at the Henle's Philadelphia virus laboratory.

Epstein reminded Denis, "As a matter of routine, every new technician starting work in the Henle laboratory has antibody tests done on a blood sample to determine past contacts with various viral agents. This is an important precaution in case a worker should accidentally be exposed to a hazardous virus during work. An acquired infection can thus be diagnosed and monitored by a rise in antibody titer to that virus."

Tony continued, "One young technician, Elaine Hutkin, became ill with fever, sore throat, and enlarged lymph nodes in the neck. She stayed home from work for six days. Shortly after returning to the lab, she developed a rash. The Henles immediately did various antibody tests to identify a possible virus. Her antibody test for the Epstein-Barr virus was positive, whereas they knew that prior to her illness, the EBV antibody was negative. In fact, they'd often used her blood as a 'negative control.' "

"She must have been one of the mere fifteen percent of Americans EBV-negative," Denis commented. "So now the Henles were observing what an acute EBV infection was like."

"Here is the most exciting part," Tony exclaimed. "Her physician diagnosed the illness as **infectious mononucleosis!** All laboratory tests for this disease were by then positive. There was no doubt that the EB virus was the cause of her illness."

Denis was amazed. "What a surprise to learn that our ubiquitous EBV is the etiologic agent of the commonly-occurring infectious mononucleosis!"

This finding automatically answered a number of puzzling questions regarding both the lymphoma and infectious mononucleosis. This latter febrile illness, nearly always self-limited, usually runs its course in two to four weeks and mostly affects adolescents or young adults. Such persons, it would soon be learned, had never had infectious mononucleosis in childhood with its consequent production of antibodies to protect against the illness in later years. A contact with the EBV in early childhood, on the other hand, usually causes no symptoms, or such mild subclinical symptoms that the disease passes unnoticed but the protective antibodies are formed. This accounts for the "silently-acquired" EBV antibodies in eighty-five percent of Americans tested.

Infectious mononucleosis, known popularly as the "kissing disease," frequents college campuses. For that reason, since 1958, Doctors Niederman and McCollum of the Yale University School of Medicine had been studying the illness in college students. As freshmen enrolled, they collected and froze serum samples from each student. If a student acquired the disease during his college days, after he became ill, a second serum sample was taken, frozen, and stored.

Now, at the Henle's request, the Yale doctors allowed the Henles to do "blind testing" on all collected paired serum samples of students who'd had the disease during their college days. Without exception, those students developing infectious mononucleosis had no EBV antibodies in their original serum samples. But their second blood specimens, taken after the illness, revealed a high titer of EBV antibodies. This was proof-positive that the EB virus caused infectious mononucleosis.

After Denis heard this most recent news regarding the EBV and infectious mononucleosis, he thought of how it related to the African scene. *It's true, we never see infectious mononucleosis among the Africans. The children there must have subclinical cases when they're very young, as all have the antibody to EBV. I suppose it's the better hygiene of the Western countries which allows a small percentage of their populations to escape coming in contact with the disease in childhood. This would account for the fifteen percent of Americans with no EBV antibodies.*

Those Western children acquiring the disease in adolescence, he reasoned, *have more severe symptoms, with a clinically recognizable disease. But if EBV can also cause the lymphoma, why do we not see more cancer, if all African children and the great majority of American children harbor EBV antibodies? Why do any children develop cancer from an EBV infection?*

These key questions made not only Burkitt, but also other investigators consider the body's immune system more seriously. Years before, Gilbert Dalldorf had suggested that a chronic malarial infection, by depressing the immune system, might be an adjunct in causing the tumor. With this new insight which infectious mononucleosis brought into the EBV picture, Denis and others also pinpointed the immune system as a possible missing-factor in the BL puzzle.

In this respect, Burkitt had found some initially unsettling new information on several of his more recent safaris in Eastern Africa. The lymphoma, which for many years he had declared to be an exclusive childhood tumor, had been found in a number of adolescents and even in a few adults.

Intensive racial and tribal distribution studies of BL throughout Uganda, led to the observation that, with the exception of three Asian Indians, all Uganda lymphoma patients had been Africans. The ratio of African to Asian cases was approximately 150 to 1, corresponding to the ratio of Africans to Asians in the general population. So race did not affect susceptibility to the tumor.

However, Denis found that immigrants coming into Uganda from two tribes of tumor-free Rwanda or Burundi, developed the tumor at an older age. About fifty percent of these patients were over fifteen years old, and twenty-six percent were over thirty. These immigrants, moving from their former, malaria-free, highland residence, presumably met an environmental agent (malaria?) at an older age when they acquired the disease in the hyperendemic malarial lowlands. **This finding of BL in older immigrants would also suggest that malaria played a part in initiating the cancer, possibly by causing an immunological depression.**

With a factor in the initiation of cancer pointing strongly to the immune system, immunologists around the world more intensely studied its possible role in all cancer-production. Thousands of scientific papers began flooding the medical literature, many using as a basis for study Burkitt's lymphoma and the Epstein-Barr virus. As a better understanding of the immune system began to unfold, this highly important body defense mechanism was found to be tremendously complicated.

Previously considered unimportant, the so-called "vestigial" organs, such as the thymus, appendix and tonsils, were already recognized as vital to body immunity. A new appreciation centered on the lymphocyte, a white blood cell, for its ability to transform or revert from a mature cell back to an immature form, a lymphoblast, capable of unlimited proliferative ability. It was in these "transformed" lymphoblasts derived from the Burkitt's tumor that Epstein had originally found the herpes-type Epstein-Barr virus.

Furthermore, lymphocytes were now being divided into two major types. The so-called "T-lymphocytes" derived their name from the *thymus* gland, where they were originally schooled for their defense functions. The "B-lymphocytes," named for their resemblance to the lymphoid cells in the Bursa of Fabricius in fowls, formed antibodies. "B-cells" in humans were thought to be schooled for their function in the bone marrow or in the lymphoid tissue of the bowel.

Investigators early found that the EB virus sought mature B-lymphocytes as "target cells." After invading the B-lymphocytes, the virus "transformed" them into immature lymphoblasts that multiplied indefinitely in tissue culture. Uninfected B-lymphocytes failed to grow or divide in culture, and died off within two or three weeks. The scientists also found that the EB virus was capable of transforming some B-lymphocytes in the living human being.

Doctor Rocchi, of the University of Rome, showed that one in five thousand B-lymphocytes in infectious mononucleosis patients was transformed, while in a healthy person, only one B-lymphocyte in ten million was transformed. **Since it was wild proliferation of transformed B-lymphoblasts that formed Burkitt's lymphoma, the disease eventually came to be classified as a "B-cell lymphoma."**

The virus infecting the B-lymphocyte produced a foreign protein "antigen" within the nucleus, the Epstein-Barr nuclear antigen. The virus also produced another "antigen" on the cell membrane. Since these virus-associated antigen-proteins were foreign to the host cell, they induced the manufacture of specific "antibodies," which, in turn, reacted with the antigen of the EB virus in an attempt to destroy it.

For years, "atypical lymphocytes" had been a diagnostic feature in the stained blood smears of patients with infectious mononucleosis. Now it was recognized that these atypical lymphocytes were actually reactive T-cells, activated to destroy the infected B-cells. Throughout the remaining life of the individual thus infected, these "memory" T-cells with cytotoxic (cell-destroying) potential, would prevent or control proliferation of the persistent EB viruses harbored in B-lymphocytes. By this means, the T-cells would keep the virus under control, producing a "latent" (inactive) state of the virus.

These facts led Burkitt and other investigators to ask, *Should these protective T-cells undergo injury and become ineffective, might not the EB infected B-cells proliferate unrestricted, leading to tumor formation?* The conclusion reached was that **suppression of the normal protective T-cell activity by chronic malaria, could thus account for the development of BL.**

Burkitt's lymphoma as well as fatal infectious mononucleosis, occurring in England and the United States could be explained by these patients' deficient immune systems. Burkitt's lymphoma would later be found in cases of hereditary immunodeficiency, as well as in patients receiving organ transplants who had been treated by drugs that suppressed the immune system. Discovering the multiple and marvelous mechanisms afforded by the immune system as protection against cancer would take thousands of scientists many years. The many-faceted Burkitt's lymphoma puzzle thus helped open new vistas in the total cancer enigma.

*****

Flipping through the May 1967 *British Medical Journal* as he sat in his London office one day, Denis found an article entitled, "Burkitt's Tumour in the West Nile District of Uganda 1961–5." *How nice! Ted finally has an article with Malcolm Pike on the "clustering" of the BL cases which he showed Hutt and me some time back. They've pointed out the unusual "epidemic" features of BL cases in these children who lived close together and developed the disease almost simultaneously. Ted is certainly to be commended for his bringing this to the attention of the rest of us.*

Not many days later in his office, Burkitt received a phone call from Dr. Richard Doll, director of the Medical Research Council's Statistical Section.

"Denis," Dr. Doll announced, "I have Captain T.L. (Peter) Cleave, a retired naval physician in my office. I think you'd be interested in meeting him."

"Tell me more," Denis invited.

"He has some different ideas about nutrition, relating it to geographical situations. Statistically, I could pull much of his work to pieces, but nonetheless I have a hunch that he might be right." Mention of the word, "geographical" aroused Burkitt's curiosity. "Send him right over," he responded, little imagining that a new horizon was about to open in his research career.

Over cups of tea that afternoon, Denis learned Peter Cleave's hypothesis. The stocky, balding man eagerly pointed out, "Many diseases most frequently found in the affluent Western countries are rare or unknown in the rural areas of the Third World. For instance," he said, "here in England we have coronary heart disease, gallstones, appendicitis, diverticular disease of the colon, diabetes, varicose veins, hemorrhoids, hiatus hernia, and peptic ulcer. But did you see these diseases in Africa?"

As Cleave mentioned the various afflictions, Burkitt ticked off each in his mind as being totally absent or rare in his African practice of medicine. Actually, he'd already found this disease difference in surgical emergencies encountered at Lira and Mulago compared with that of his brother Robin's practice in England. In fact, back in 1952, Denis and Robin had published a paper noting these disease differences in the two cultures.

Gradually, Cleave approached the main focus of his hypothesis. He shifted uneasily in his chair. "There are associations among these Western-type diseases," he stressed. "Not only do they have similar geographical and socioeconomic distributions, but they also tend to occur together in the same patients. These Western-type diseases must therefore share some causative factors," he concluded.

This reasoning sounded familiar to Denis, for ten years previously he had thought of a "common cause"

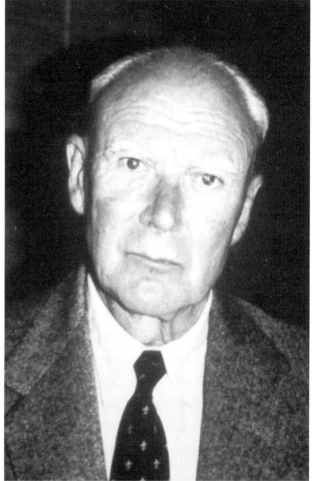

Nutritional investigator, Capt. T. L. (Peter) Cleave.

when finding multiple tumors spread throughout the bodies of children with BL. His interest aroused, Denis asked, "So what do you consider is the common cause of all these diseases you've just named?"

"I've come to the conclusion," Cleave said, "that these afflictions have emerged with the adoption of a new culture by the Western world, and represent a maladaptation to the new environment."

"Precisely what change in the culture?" Burkitt probed, crossing his arms over his chest.

Cleave handed Denis his book. "I have here my book, in which I explain my ideas."

155

Denis looked at the title, *Coronary Heart Disease, Diabetes and the Saccharine Disease*, and said, "I suppose by 'saccharine' you mean that these Western diseases are caused by an excessive consumption of sugar."

"The refining process," Cleave explained, "extracts sugar in a concentrated, fiber-free form from either the cane or beet, and overconsumption of refined sugar leads, in time, to all these diseases."

As he turned the pages of the book, Denis was amazed by the number of his references and asked, "Tell me, just how have you collected all your data?"

Cleave leaned forward in his earnestness, saying, "I've spent many years working on the project. Actually I've written in longhand some twenty thousand letters to doctors all over the world."

Denis raised his eyebrows at this figure. But Cleave continued, "From those who responded, as well as from my own observations, I've drawn my conclusions. I'm well aware that these ideas are not acceptable to conventional medical thought." Pointing to the cover again, he drew Burkitt's attention to the names of the authors. "You'll notice that Dr. G.D. Campbell in South Africa was a co-author with me of the book. He's a diabetes specialist."

Denis stood up, closing the interview with a final comment. "Let me read your book so that I can better understand your position. I'll get in touch with you again."

After the Captain left, Denis thumbed through the book carefully, reasoning that the man's clear thinking and courageous challenging of present medical concepts were appealing. He noted that Dr. Richard Doll, who had sent Cleave to him, had written the Foreword to the book:

> Whether the predictions that Surgeon Captain Cleave and Dr. Campbell make in this book will prove to be correct remains to be seen; but if only a small part of them do, the authors will have made a bigger contribution to medicine than most university departments or medical research units make in the course of a generation.

That's quite a statement by Doll! thought Denis. As he read the book more carefully, he found Cleave's main hypothesis was, as Cleave had stated, that many diseases of the Western culture were directly due to the refining of carbohydrate foods, incriminating sugar as the main villain. The captain had underscored that these diseases were now equally common in both black and white Americans but rare in native Africans. He concluded that the diseases were primarily environmental rather than genetic. Burkitt found Cleave's hypothesis fairly in harmony with his own experience and initially accepted it all with the proviso that it be proven by investigation.

At this time, Burkitt was occasionally making surgical rounds in both British and American hospitals. He couldn't avoid contrasting, as he had years before, the common operations in Western hospitals for appendicitis, diverticular disease, gallbladder disease, hiatus hernia, and hemorrhoids. He knew that these diseases were absent in rural African facilities. Ian McAdam, he remembered, used to tell the African medical students, "Don't ever diagnose appendicitis unless the patient speaks English." This was to emphasize that appendicitis was only associated with Western culture, education, and city dwelling. *What dietary changes in these Africans accompanied their cultural changes?* Denis wondered.

Burkitt felt, at this stage, like someone who was climbing a mountain and at the summit, having reached the skyline, sees a whole new panorama spread before him. He realized he was possibly the only man alive in a position to check out Cleave's ideas, for he had built up a network, mainly of mission hospitals in Africa, which were reporting on cancer patients every month. He might widen his questionnaire to inquire regarding appendicitis, gall stones, diverticular disease, bowel cancer, diabetes, and the rest of these "Western diseases."

His interest aroused, he began to read and research in the field of nutrition. Cleave, he found, was not the first to suspect refined food as a culprit in causing certain diseases. A Dr. T. R. Allinson in 1880 had written:

> One great curse of this country is constipation of the bowels which is caused in great measure by white bread. From this constipation comes piles, varicose veins, headaches, miserable feelings, dullness and other ailments. Separating the bran from the flour may be said to have come into fashion at the beginning of this century and as a consequence pill factories arose and are now an almost necessary part of the State. Would you banish the pill box from your private cupboard? Then you must drive white bread from your table.

Interesting that Allinson mentioned a relationship between bran and both piles and varicose veins, thought Denis. He laughed as he read that the poor doctor had lost his medical license, being accused of malpractice for selling whole wheat bread. The brass plate on his office bore the title, "Dr. T.R. Allinson, Ex-M.R.C.P."

Although the many new scientific developments around the world in various aspects of the Burkitt lymphoma-EB virus problem still fascinated Denis, here was an entirely new area of geographical medicine. Was it providential that he now had just the right African hospital system, all in place, to compare diet and disease and prove Cleave either right or wrong?

13

TABOO STUDIES

Burkitt admitted to himself that Captain Cleave's book dealing with the "saccharine disease" had aroused his interest. Although he couldn't agree that sugar was the main culprit in the causation of many so-called Western diseases, he thoroughly agreed with Cleave's other ideas. He had rarely, if ever, seen diseases of the Western culture in the rural African population. Never in "up-country" Africans had he operated on cases of acute appendicitis, gallstones, diverticular disease of the bowel, or hemorrhoids. He felt it was time to get in touch with Cleave for another conversation.

This time, Cleave came loaded with other books he had written, on peptic ulcer and varicose veins. "I've published these at my own expense," he said. "The medical profession," he complained, "doesn't listen to me. Consequently, I can't find a publisher for my research."

"In reading through your book, " Burkitt began, as they sat together in his office, "I note that you stress sugar as the main cause of these diseases because of the refining process. But what about the fiber removed at the same time?" Denis knew that millers, in grinding grain for wheat flour, removed the bran, disposing of it by feeding it to animals. He also knew, from his recent reading, that few doctors appreciated the value of bran and fiber, the indigestible cell walls of plant food. Bran lacked nutritional value, they said, and some physicians considered it too coarse for humans.

"When I was in the navy during the war," Cleave confessed, "I treated constipated sailors by giving them bran. Bran may have a role, but I think that sugar is the greater culprit," he declared.

Testing him a bit more, Burkitt said, "There are other food components, you know, such as fat. What do you think about fat in the diet?"

"I don't think that fat plays any appreciable role. It's the carbohydrate refining process and sugar in particular which give the problem." Cleave was dogmatic.

Burkitt tried again to find common ground. "I appreciate what you said in your book about spending our medical resources on drug and surgical treatment in the West, rather than on prevention of disease. If it's wrong eating habits that are killing us by causing many lethal diseases, making proper dietary changes would certainly be an economical form of therapy." Any good modality that saved money always rated high in Denis's opinion. "I'll work with you, Peter," he said, rising from his chair to indicate the end of the interview.

In 1967, when Burkitt first conversed with Cleave, he was receiving monthly cancer figures from more than 150 hospitals in the Third World. These were mainly mission facilities, not only in Africa, but some also in Southeast Asia and South America.

It seems to me, Denis thought, *Cleave may have some ideas worth investigating, and since I'm probably the only person in a position to test them, I'll just make out a new questionnaire to spell out these Western diseases and ask how often they're seen in the participating hospitals.*

As Denis thought about the possible role of various food components, he always came back to fiber. *Cleave admitted giving bran for constipation. Adequate fiber in the diet certainly prevents constipation, and might not constipation itself contribute to some of these disorders, like hemorrhoids, diverticular disease and hiatus hernia?*

He decided to look further into the history of fiber. But for his search of medical literature in the *Cumulative Indices Medicus*, he was unable to find "fiber" listed. He found "fiber optics," but no "dietary fiber" category. "Constipation" proved a more fruitful heading. To his surprise, he discovered that even Hippocrates, the "father of Western medicine," had commented on the laxative properties of coarse flour over that of fine flour.

In his historical research on constipation, Denis found that a famous late 19th century British surgeon, Sir Arbuthnot Lane, had even done radical surgery with removal of the colon for what he considered "stagnation" of the large bowel content. Fortunately, Lane later discovered that severe constipation could be alleviated very simply with miller's bran. He began preaching this doctrine far and wide, but unfortunately, his simple antidote failed to become popular.

An old friend of Lane's, fellow surgeon, Dr. J. H. Kellogg, chief physician at the famous Battle Creek Sanitarium in Michigan, joined Lane in espousing the idea of "autointoxication." Elie Metchnikoff, a Russian chemist, had put forth a theory— that the body absorbed decomposing food residues in the colon as toxic waste products. To prevent

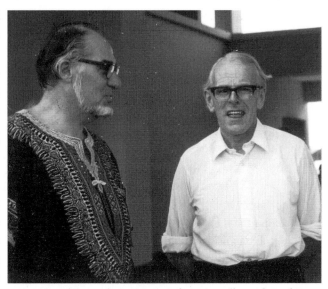

Ray Knighton, administrator of M.A.P. talks with Burkitt.

this "autointoxication," Kellogg became convinced that a bowel movement following each meal was nature's way of preserving good health. He opposed all use of laxatives and instead recommended increased consumption of wheat bran, vegetables and water.

Kellogg, in the early 1900's, frequently quoted Sylvester Graham, for whom "Graham crackers" were named, another pioneer in nutrition, who insisted that housewives make bread from whole wheat or "graham" flour. This unrefined flour contained bran and germ elements as well as the starchy components of wheat.

Denis entered his new area of research slowly, for his main activity and interest still lay with the lymphoma problem. In mid-October of 1967, he and Olive flew to Boston, where he lectured at both Tufts and Harvard Universities. He also attended a major lymphoma conference being held at Ann Arbor, Michigan, for which he had prepared a paper. He caught the attention of the participants by surprisingly *not* lecturing on BL, but rather on fiber and Western diseases!

While attending the conference, Denis practiced what he preached by bringing a bag of bran to breakfast and sprinkling it generously over his cereal. Of course Burkitt's purpose in this act was twofold—not only for his own health, but to arouse further interest in fiber by any who might observe him. Dr. Vincent de Vitas, for one, especially noted Burkitt's practice. He was to play an important future role in the distribution of cancer research money in the United States as director of the National Cancer Institute.

While in Michigan, Denis and Olive visited again with their good friends, the Blocksmas; in Chicago, they once more stayed with Ray Knighton, who was soon to have a part in Denis's nutritional research program. Following further lectures in Washington D.C. and New York, the Burkitts returned to England. By mid-November, Denis was off again for two days, this time lecturing at a Paris conference.

*****

By early 1968, a cancer unit in Accra had been named for Denis, the Burkitt Tumor Center. In East Africa, the Burkitt Lymphoma Center now occupied some of the older buildings at the Mulago Hospital. In February, exciting information on the relation of malaria to BL was at last emerging. Several investigators were studying a chronic malarial depression of the immune system, associated with *Plasmodium falciparum*, as a step in the development of the tumor.

Writing various lymphoma papers, as well as having consultations with Doll, Hutt and Wright, occupied Denis's spring months. May 18 he received a pleasant and certainly unexpected honor, the Arnott Gold Medal. The Irish hospitals and Medical Schools Association presented this award for his work on BL.

On a transatlantic flight to New York, June 7, he had the unusual experience of being the sole tourist passenger on a Boeing 707. How this happened, the stewardesses couldn't explain, but they gave him royal treatment. Being ever the photographer, he took a picture of all the empty seats to record the occasion and authenticate his strange story. Lectures in New York, Houston, and Los Angeles occupied a weeklong trip. But his most important stop was in Chicago to elicit Ray Knighton's help. Friend Ralph Blocksma had suggested more than once that the Medical Assistance Program (M.A.P), of which he had been president since its inception, could be of great help to Denis's nutritional research.

This organization gathered excessive stocks of unused drugs and medical equipment from various firms and sent them free to more than 1,000 mission hospitals in the Third World. The U.S. government recognized the philanthropic value of this totally nonprofit, multimillionaire dollar enterprise, even offering to pay freight charges to any country exempting these gifts from customs duty. Leaders of several Third World countries had honored Knighton, the executive-director, for his vision and M.A.P. contributions to their rural hospitals. In the future, the American Medical Association would also extend to Knighton its highest award given to a nonmedical man.

Since M.A.P. regularly sent shipments to far-flung mission hospitals, Denis asked if a simple nutritional questionnaire could be enclosed in each shipment. He felt that the recipients of the free supplies would be happy to answer a survey concerning the occurrence of Western-type diseases in their areas. Ray readily agreed to send out Burkitt's nutritional inquiry as soon as he could prepare it.

By early 1969, Denis was fully involved with the epidemiological studies on Western diseases. He had already received substantial replies to his first question-naire sent to the 150 mission hospitals. There was, as he had anticipated, a resounding "never" or "rarely seen" to the query regarding the presence of Western diseases in these rural hospitals.

*****

One fact Burkitt realized he needed to establish was the transit-times of food passage through the alimentary tracts of various cultural groups who ate widely differing diets. Did a high-fiber diet cause more rapid passage of food through the gastrointestinal tract?

He began this study on a willing subject, a vegetarian whose diet was high in fiber. The friend swallowed, one after another, twenty-four barium-impregnated plastic pellets. Then, over a four-day period, he collected each stool into separately labeled plastic bags, noting date and time of evacuation. The stools were weighed and x-rayed to determine the number of x-ray-opaque pellets found in each. In this manner, the transit time of food residue through the gastrointestinal tract was determined.

Burkitt's June 20 diary entry stated: "Spent considerable time at home with family labeling plastic bags for bowel transit studies." His family, as always, was involved with even the menial aspects of his research. On July 4, another entry indicated his determination for family involvement in the project. "Finished bowel transit-times on family. This is necessary before going to others." When home in England, Denis repeatedly did these bowel studies among various socioeconomic groups, gathering important data as to their dietary habits.

On one occasion, in order to collect specimens from boys in an English public school, he first lectured them on diet and health, explaining how eating mostly *unrefined* food was important to avoid serious disease in their adult lives. Then he personally went to the school for the next five mornings, collecting stool specimens. After weighing all the plastic-bagged specimens, he carried them by train to London for x-raying in a hospital next to his office. After eighty percent of the swallowed barium-opaque pellets showed up by x-ray in the stool specimens, the tests were complete, and transit-times were recorded.

After all his efforts, he had been able to enlist a mere thirty brave volunteers at the school, of whom only twenty actually finished the test. He would find that compiling transit-time information on Western children was one of his most difficult tasks, for the youngsters frequently forgot to save their stool specimens.

While on his next safari to East Africa, Denis talked to the head master at the Budo Mission school, where his friend, Dick Drown, had worked. There he recruited twenty-six student volunteers. The results were very different from those of English school boys. From this small beginning, Denis continued his stool studies on each subsequent African safari.

*****

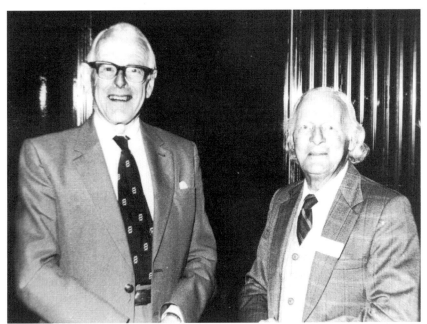

Burkitt with Dr. Alec Walker in South Africa.

On a trip to the United States in May 1969, Burkitt lectured at the Cook County Hospital in Chicago. Since this venerable facility had records going back for scores of years, he wanted to find prevalent diseases of black Americans before they had adopted affluent Western eating habits and life-styles. As Cleave had pointed out, black Americans now suffered from the same Western diseases as their Caucasian American neighbors. It was as he expected, over the decades there had been a gradually rising incidence of the Western diseases in black Americans.

At a later time, when lecturing on fiber in the United States, Denis suggested that someone in his audience ought to do a study contrasting transit-times of current black and white Americans. Philadelphia University Medical School's Professor of Surgery, Dr. Harry Goldsmith, accepted the challenge and conducted such studies on his medical students. He found no significant differences in bowel transit-times among his black and white students.

In the summer of 1969, the Burkitts took a much deserved respite. In company with their Christian friends from Africa, Jack and Beryl Darling, they boarded a ship to Oslo for the third International Conference of Christian Physicians and Dentists. Denis had always been active in the organization, frequently holding a major office. It was a joyful time of reunion with old friends, and while in Oslo, they witnessed the historic landing of men on the moon.

Saying goodbye to Olive in the Reading station in August, Denis was off on a month-long trip to Uganda, Kenya, Tanzania and South Africa to engage in several safaris. This time he had a greater focus on his new nutritional interest. In Durban, South Africa, Denis met and conversed at length with Dr. G. D. Campbell, the diabetes specialist who was listed as Cleave's co-author. Campbell's grandfather, ironically, had been the first to import sugar cane into Natal. Now sugar, the country's major export, was being berated as a health hazard by Campbell's own grandson!

Burkitt also got to know Dr. Alec Walker on this trip, initiating a close and lasting friendship. Walker had come to South Africa in 1938 after completing his biochemistry training in England. Now that Denis was newly focusing on nutritional problems, his inquiries concerned fiber.

"I understand that you've had an interest in nutrition for some time," Burkitt began, as he approached Walker on the subject.

"That's right. It's been sort of a hobby of mine for about thirty years," Walker admitted, with a friendly smile. "My introduction to the subject involved work with African prisoners during the second World war."

"I'd like to know more details, because, as a surgeon I've only recently become aware of a fiber problem in the diet," Burkitt told him.

"You know how it was during the war with the wheat shortage, not only in Europe, but also here in South Africa," Walker began. "The government wanted the millers to extract less bran so that wheat supplies would stretch farther. But they soon found that whole wheat bread, with its high bran content, was relatively more laxative than refined white bread. Consequently they feared that eating whole wheat bread would lead to excessive calcium loss in the stool.

"Since my doctoral degree was in biochemistry," Walker explained, "I was asked to determine calcium in the stools of both white volunteers and black prisoners. The two groups first ate white bread, followed a week later by whole wheat bread. It was my job to determine the relative calcium losses in both the Whites and Blacks on the two diets."

"I'm curious to know what you found," Denis said.

"Initially, there was some increased calcium loss when the two groups went on whole wheat bread," Walker said. "But, very shortly, a calcium balance occurred. However, as I continued the studies, I noticed a marked difference in stool weights of the two groups. The African prisoners on a native, totally unrefined diet had stools three times the weight of white volunteers, who ate a typically refined European diet."

"That's exactly what I've been finding, comparing the stool weights of rural Africans with those of English school boys. The Africans have much larger, softer stools, and I've attributed this to the higher fiber content of the native diets," Denis said. "But don't let me interrupt you. I'm very interested."

"I next became curious as to the time it took for food to pass through the alimentary tract. I wondered if there would be a difference in the two groups." Walker continued his account. "So I prepared food coloring in capsules and gave these to the volunteers, noting the time of administration. Then I observed the time when the dye appeared in the stools. Just as I'd thought, the bowel transit-time was much more rapid in the Africans on their unrefined diet. These African prisoners were never constipated!" Walker shifted his weight from one leg to the other as he talked.

"Another fact I learned from the prison doctors was that the Africans never had appendicitis." Burkitt nodded at this last bit of information. "By then," the biochemist added, "I was pretty certain that the lack of both constipation and appendicitis was due to their increased fiber consumption."

"Have you done other studies?" Denis asked, feeling quite certain that he had.

"The absence of appendicitis in the prisoners made me wonder about other illnesses as well. So I studied different disease patterns among the Whites, Blacks, Coloreds and Indians living in South Africa. I cataloged their differing diets and found appendicitis thirty times more common among Whites than Blacks." Walker recalled the statistics. "Few Africans had diabetes, gallstones or obesity, which were frequent in the Whites. It was only as the Blacks became urbanized and began eating refined foods that they suffered from the same diseases as the Whites."

"So you've found no differences attributable to race?" Denis asked.

"None," Walker said. "Another disease I found only in urban populations was colon cancer. I feel that this cancer is also associated with a fiber-depleted diet."

"You're certainly right," Denis admitted. "Cancer of the colon is an unknown disease among the more primitive Third World people. There's got to be a good reason for this."

"I believe that the increased length of time that food remains in the bowel in a fiber-deficient, constipated person, allows more opportunity for ingested carcinogens to act on the lining cells of the bowel," Walker explained.

Burkitt agreed. "Cancer of the colon is another disease that would fit into the classification of Western diseases. Peter Cleave introduced me to the concept of a refined diet and Western diseases. Perhaps you've heard of him?"

"Yes, Campbell showed me his book," Walker said. "But he believes that sugar is the cause of all these diseases and scarcely mentions the loss of fiber in the refining process."

"We've had quite a few discussions on this point," Denis said, laughing, "but I don't know that I'm convincing him at all. He's a good man, very dedicated to this work, and certainly an example of untiring industry. He's had an enormous impact on my life!" With this final remark, the two men parted. Denis had learned a great deal from his conversation with the kindly Walker.

On this same South African trip, Denis determined to look up Drs. Anthony and Maggy Barker at a mission hospital in adjacent Zululand. Cleave had quoted these missionaries, working in a remote area, who reported the rarity of coronary heart disease, varicose veins, hemorrhoids and still other Western diseases. The Barkers welcomed Burkitt and invited him to attend the before-breakfast ward rounds conducted daily. Dr. Anthony, a surgeon, and Dr. Maggy, a general physician, confirmed what Cleave had recorded in his book. They rarely saw Western diseases in their part of rural Africa.

Denis wondered, *Why is it, with all these well-qualified doctors individually working on the idea of fiber-depleted diets as causing Western diseases, that the medical profession in general doesn't know of their findings? If doctors have heard theories regarding diet-related disease, why do some of them consider these conscientious, medical fact-finders mere "quacks" or "food-fanatics?"* Again, Denis felt it was time to speak out and let the world know the truth. By now he had adequate facts to back up the fiber theories.

The trip had been most profitable, and on his return to England, he plunged into his writing and research with ever-increasing eagerness. On September 2 he wrote in his diary: "Cleave called. He mentioned his controversy with Campbell, his co-author." This was news, for Denis had just met Campbell in South Africa, who hadn't hinted of any problem. Somehow, jealousies were involved. Denis thoroughly appreciated the lonely years of effort that Cleave had put into his theory, and he determined anew always to give him full credit when referring to his findings.

That September, Burkitt flew to Sao Paulo, Brazil, where a conference sponsored by the American Cancer Society was being held. In his lecture, he spoke on Burkitt's lymphoma. However, privately he mentioned to one of the senior executives of the Society the work which Walker had done on the possible relationship between fiber-deficient diets and colon cancer. As a result of this conversation, Denis was invited to speak at the next American Cancer Society meeting to be held in San Diego, California, several months later.

While on this, his first trip to South America, he took the opportunity to visit Belem, at the mouth of the Amazon and learn as much as he could regarding the geographical pathology of the region. His return trip included a stop at the Sloane-Kettering Institute in New York, where he was presented with the Katherine Berkan Judd Award for his work in chemotherapy on Burkitt's lymphoma in African children.

Denis's interests were always divided and full. Besides medicine, there were his Christian endeavors and also vital, his home and family. In November, he and Olive had a meeting of friends in their living room to discuss the formation of a Bible-study group. They decided not to invite a vicar to attend, thereby insuring more spontaneity of those present. On December 31, he ended 1969 with this note in his diary: "Eleven for supper. Ten for night. Cassy made supper. Olive always does an enormous amount of entertaining."

✷✷✷✷✷

Continuing his interest in bowel transit-times, Denis met a senior doctor in the British navy medical services with whom he was able to arrange for studies on sailors at sea. On shipboard, the sailors' lives were fairly sedentary and they ate standard ship's food, a typically refined fare.

When home from foreign travel during these years, he continued to conduct the bowel studies among various socioeconomic groups. He wanted enough evidence to support his theses, regardless of what questions or criticisms might surface.

Stool studies in Britain, he was finding, were stereotyped: small, 80–120 gram (3–4 oz.), firm-to-hard stools with transit-times varying from three to five days. Elderly nursing home patients had transit-times sometimes exceeding two weeks. In contrast, stool studies in adult rural South Africans showed an average daily stool weight of 300 to 500 grams (9–16 oz.), with bowel transit-times averaging thirty hours. White South Africans, by comparison, had 100–150 gram (3–5 oz.) stools with an average transit time of seventy hours, comparable to the British and American. Tests in India and Southeast Asia produced results intermediate between the African and British figures.

As Burkitt lectured more and more on the subject of fiber, he naturally needed to include his stool data. Thus, to subtly introduce the "delicate" subject, he frequently used Lord Byron's ditty. It was said to have been written on Byron's lavatory wall in Newstead Abbey, near Nottingham:

> Cloaca Goddess of this place,
> Look on thy suppliant with a smiling face.
> Soft and obedient may his motions flow,
> Not rashly swift or obstinately slow.

Talking about stools in public was, at first, met with a lifted eyebrow. Stools were considered a "taboo" subject. But Denis threw away all caution by arousing interest among both his medical colleagues and his nonmedical audiences. Often in referring to his findings, he maintained that "Britain (or America) is a constipated nation." Taking a humorous tack, he shockingly projected on the screen a colored slide of a large, poorly-formed stool photographed near the path in an African village. He

167

contrasted this with a picture of the small, hard balls of feces typical of the Western world. "A 'normal stool' in a person who eats a high-fiber diet should float in water," he advised. "On such a diet, one should not be surprised to pass foot-long stools more than once a day!"

To spice up his lectures and to show that his observations were not new, he used excerpts from a book published in 1723 in Dublin entitled, *Human Odure*. It was authored by a mysterious "Dr. S...t." The book was a treatise on human excreta as observed by the author and classified into five categories. Category one—the ideal, he described in this way (in old English, the "f" = "s"):

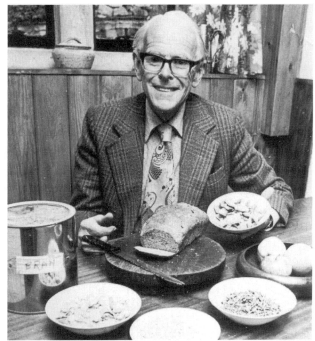

Burkitt demonstrates high-fiber foods.

> ...refembling a boy's top revers'd. The diftinguishing characteristik of this kind of evacuation is that it rifes with a broad bafis, and terminates with a narrow apex; under this denomination is comprehended those formed like an obelifk, chefhine hat, sugarloaf, a pyramid or Portugal pear.

As Denis read a further description of the ideal 1723 stool, he decided it was also the ideal for the 1970's.

> There are always generated in a robuft ftrong body and give us some indications of a well ton'd fet of intestines, to be met moftly in plow'd field, high roads and fometimes in meadows.

The mysterious author's fifth category description fit quite accurately current Western stools.

...voided in small, firm, round, diftinct balls, buttons or bullets.
I have obferved thefe species to flourifh moftly about colleges,
schools, and moft places of publick education.

Obviously the diet of the educated, wealthy, upper classes was more constipating than that of the common laborer or farmer!

The anonymous name of the author, "Dr. S---t," on the title page of the old volume so intrigued Denis that, when in Edinburgh, he took the book to a dealer in antique literature. The gentleman searched through old catalogs and, to Denis' delight, identified the writer. He was Dean Jonathan Swift, author of *Gulliver's Travels*, and a most illustrious graduate of Denis's own university, Trinity College, Dublin.

*****

In preparing his lecture for the American Cancer Society's conference in San Diego, Denis spent considerable time outlining the geographical distribution of colon cancer, especially in Africa. He used Walker's fiber-depleted-diet hypothesis as a major factor responsible for the growing number of bowel cancers in the Western world and other prosperous societies. These fiber-deficient diets emphasized meat, white bread, dairy products and rich desserts.

Most cancer researchers currently considered fat the prime suspect in bowel cancer, with animal protein a second possibility. They looked at foods *consumed* in the diet, while Denis and Walker suggested dietary fiber, as a *missing constituent* in the Western menu.

Press coverage of the cancer meeting immediately picked up the fiber story and gave widespread exposure to the idea that dietary fiber protected from the increasingly prevalent colon cancer. But there was also much skepticism within the medical profession. Burkitt's paper on the subject, published in the *Cancer* journal in 1971, gave the idea further publicity.

The fiber theory had been launched. Burkitt, with his high reputation in the scientific world, could expect at least a listening audience. He acted as a spokesman for his friends, Alec Walker, Peter Cleave, and later, Hugh Trowell, in promoting an all-important attack on Western diseases. At this time he mused, *Had the B-lymphocytes in the immune system been discovered a few years earlier, the African lymphoma would never have been called "Burkitt's lymphoma" but rather a "B-cell lymphoma." And if there'd been no "Burkitt's lymphoma," I would be considered just another food crank!*

This fact became evident following his address on fiber and Western diseases to the Edinburgh Medical Society, the oldest medical student body in the world. Olive had accompanied him, and after the meeting, a student, not realizing she was Mrs. Burkitt, said to her, "That was a good talk, but no one except Burkitt could have gotten away with saying what he did!"

Where else would his influence make an impact?

14

FORTUITOUS CONTACTS

With enthusiasm and skill, Burkitt attacked the nutritional problem of Western diseases even as he had previously attacked the African lymphoma. The titles of his 1970 scientific papers betrayed his shifting interest, with nine of his fourteen medical articles that year, diet-oriented. There were, for example: *"Diet and Non-infective Disease of the Large Bowel,"* and *"An Epidemiological Approach to Gastrointestinal Cancer."*

His newly sparked preference for preventive medicine rather than the standard therapy appeared in other titles: *"Limitations of Scientific Medicine," "Are Our Commonest Killing Diseases Preventable?"* and *"Disease and Death from Avoidable Causes."*

Even though therapeutic medicine is necessary, he thought, *how much better to prevent disease and avoid the necessity of costly treatment.* He now regretted the fact that his twenty years in Africa had made no impact on the total health of the country, for his time had been devoted to salvaging individual cases. He would come to realize that Western countries have directed ninety-nine percent of medical effort toward attempted cure. Only a tiny one percent of modern medical attention has been devoted to the prevention of disease.

Beginning at this period in his mounting nutritional campaign, he aimed his guns in a humorous way at his own fellow physicians. He wanted to arouse them to see the health benefits for their patients in preventing avoidable disease. Burkitt recognized that medical training overemphasized curative medicine, with its inherent personal financial gains. Illustrating his argument, he often stated, "At a relatively small cost of three hundred million dollars (one-eightieth the cost of putting a man on the moon), smallpox can be eradicated from the face of the earth. In 1967 there were two million deaths from smallpox, whereas simple prevention by mass worldwide vaccination would save millions of lives at a relatively insignificant cost per person." Smallpox has since been eliminated from the globe by this very means.

In March 1970, Olive accompanied Denis on another multipurpose trip to Africa, this being her first return since their 1966 departure. One reason for the trip was the conferral on Burkitt of an honorary Doctorate in Science by the University of East Africa. In tandem with the ceremony was a special conference in Kampala commemorating the centennial of Sir Albert Cook's birth. Sir Albert, who died in 1951 in Uganda at the age of eighty-one, had been the country's most famous doctor and the founder of the Mengo Hospital. Mulago Hospital had been a spinoff facility, started as a venereal disease clinic when Cook was campaigning to eradicate a syphilis plague that was wiping out the African populace.

Also invited to attend the conference, at government expense, was Dr. Hugh Trowell, who had served in Kenya and Uganda from 1930 to 1960 and had been Sir Albert's personal physician during the later years of his life.

On this centennial occasion, Prof. Michael Hutt gave the Fifth Albert Cook Memorial Lecture. Hutt would himself be shortly leaving Africa, returning to St. Thomas's University in London to become the professor of geographical pathology. After his lecture, as a demonstration of their love and esteem, the African medical students honored him with gifts.

For this event, Burkitt decided that his lecture invitation would cover a subject different from the expected topic, the lymphoma. By now having gathered considerable data in his nutritional surveys, he consequently elected to speak on diet and disease relationships in Western and Third World cultures. He was quite unaware of Hugh Trowell's presence in the large audience. At the conclusion of the talk, Trowell immediately pressed forward to speak with his old friend.

"Denis," he exclaimed, excitedly, "I appreciate the concepts you're proposing. You remember that nutrition was my special concern for years. I think you'd be interested in seeing my book, *Non-infective Diseases In Africa*, which I wrote about ten years ago."

"Good to see you again, Hugh!" Denis enthusiastically shook hands with his old friend. "No, I hadn't heard of this book, but I certainly do recall that you were always fascinated by nutrition."

"The book had very little circulation. But at that time, among other things, I'd gone through all the African literature to compile a list of diseases never seen in Africa though common in Western countries." Highly pleased with Burkitt's lecture, Trowell said, "My list of diseases and those you've just mentioned are nearly identical."

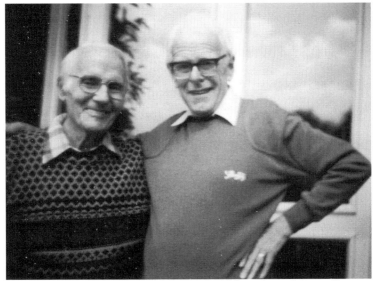

Burkitt renews acquaintance with old friend, Hugh Trowell.

"Can I get a copy of your book, Hugh?" Denis asked, and in almost the same breath inquired, "Where do you place the blame for the initiation of these diseases? I mentioned in my lecture that Peter Cleave has done years of study on the subject and that he adheres strongly to a refined carbohydrate, specifically sugar, as the culprit."

"I had hinted at the beneficial attributes of dietary cellulose in my book, but the whole subject needs more intensive study." Hugh could hardly contain his enthusiasm, for at last there were others, including his good friend, Burkitt, who were finally looking seriously at a faulty dietary to explain many common diseases of modern society.

"Are you still pastoring a church, Hugh?" Denis asked, knowing that after leaving Kampala years before, Trowell had become a minister.

"No, I've just recently retired. I was previously the pastor of a village church in Stratford-Subcastle," Trowell replied.

"We must get together for another talk, Hugh, and I hope you'll bring along a copy of your book," Denis said, giving his old friend a hug as they parted.

During this same trip to Kampala, Denis learned that Dr. Ted Dimmock, who was temporarily filling in at the Mengo Hospital, also believed in the efficacy of fiber in preventing constipation. Burkitt determined, while there, to have a chat with him. Responding to his inquiries, Dimmock said that in 1936, for his M.D. degree, he'd written a thesis on the use of miller's bran in treatment of constipation to avoid hemorrhoids. At that time, he too had weighed and analyzed many stools.

Denis now began to feel it providential that he was meeting so many different persons who had worked on nutritional problems. In fact, many years later he would state, "I was quite unconscious of the hand of God at the time various opportunities opened, and only in looking back could I discern how wonderfully I was being led. Some would call such openings 'coincidence,' 'luck,' 'serendipity,' 'good fortune,' 'chance,' but I have always been convinced of God's providential leading."

While the Burkitts were in Africa, a safari, of course, was included. This time Denis and Olive traveled to Karapokot, a northern district populated by pastoral nomadic tribes. In cooperation with a local missionary physician, Dr. David Webster, they collected many stool specimens from these tribes people for transit-time determinations. Persuading the goat-skin-clad natives to swallow the barium-opaque pellets and then to save their stool specimens was no easy task. Denis could read their thoughts from the amused, unbelieving expressions on their faces, which said: "What is so valuable about our stools that these crazy foreigners put them in those clear bags and carry them away?"

Before the Burkitts left the primitive bush hospital, Webster presented them with a hand-carved wooden stool made by a local tribesman. Attached to it was a note: "In remembrance of your interest in Karapokot stools." Denis's good sense of humor carried him through many occasions, such as this, while he collected his data. His next destination with the labeled plastic bags was the Mulago Hospital, 300 miles away, where he would determine the elimination time of the x-ray-opaque pellets.

One more occasion needed to be celebrated before they returned to England. A new, expanded orthopedic center for the construction of leg prostheses was to open in Kampala. Trained technicians were now making increasingly more functional and sophisticated appliances since the days, twenty years earlier, when Denis had initiated the manufacture of his first crude artificial limbs and leg braces.

A few days after their return home, Judy developed acute appendicitis and underwent surgery. *How ironic!* thought Denis. *Here I am studying the causes of Western diseases, including appendicitis, and my own daughter gets the disease.*

To his way of thinking, appendicitis was simply "constipation" of the appendix. If the normally-soft fecal content of the appendix became hard, a small rocklike ball called a "fecalith" formed in the proximal end, interfering with the emptying of fecal material from the appendix into the colon. The resultant swelling of the appendix interfered with the blood circulation in its wall, causing gangrene, bacterial invasion, and pus formation inside. Such an appendix could burst if not removed.

Denis had been reading in medical literature concerning this very disease. Dr. Arthur Rendle Short of Bristol University, in 1920 argued that the main cause of appendicitis was the "considerable removal of cellulose from food." He linked the refining of wheat grain to appendicitis and especially condemned the growing popularity of white flour.

One of Dr. Short's surgical duties was to provide medical care to 1,000 orphans. This enabled him to compare the rarity of appendicitis among the whole-grain-eating orphans with its prevalence among the cake-and-pastry-eating public schoolboys. Denis agreed that Dr. Short's hypothesis was surely correct.

As a result of Judy's appendicitis, Denis decided that the Burkitts must be a rather typical Western family, for in spite of eating a fairly prudent diet, they had not been exempt from acquiring a Western disease.

*****

The Burkitt household in 1970 experienced an ever-increasing tempo of life, if that was possible. An important entry in his diary was made on April 16: "Our book, *Burkitt's Lymphoma* (co-authored with Dennis Wright), started six years ago, appeared today. To God be the glory!" With some satisfaction, Denis examined the book's spectacular dust-cover, picturing the characteristic lymphoma cells. They had dedicated the volume to "The Up-Country Doctors in Africa." Its foreword, written by Sir Harold Himsworth, spelled out a provocative truth.

No explanation of cancer, or of the normal mechanism the disturbance of which underlies this, will ever be adequate unless it satisfactorily accounts for this particular tumor [Burkitt's lymphoma], **its distribution, its age incidence, its response to therapy and its relation to other diseases. In a sense, this tumor may well prove to be something of a Rosetta Stone.**

*****

In his diary on April 20, Burkitt wrote: "Long talk with Cleave." He was having frequent conversations with the captain who had proved quite intractable, holding firmly to his saccharine theory. It seemed that he scarcely listened when Denis attempted to suggest fiber-depletion and excessive fat consumption as alternative causes of Western diseases. A further diary entry on April 22 concerned Judy's future: "Philip Howard came to supper." On May 28, Denis recorded: "Saw my biography by Bernard Glemser for the first time, *Mr. Burkitt and Africa.*"

In spite of his packed schedule, Burkitt annually lectured at a refresher course taken by medical missionaries from all over the world. He used these occasions to talk with them and gain information concerning diseases seen in their practices. Also, twice a year he lectured at the Tropical Disease Hospital in Liverpool and at the School of Tropical Medicine in London. In both places he was able to meet and ask questions of doctors from various Third World countries. These physicians were able to verify his growing statistics showing the absence of Western diseases in underdeveloped countries.

In June, he made another trip to South Africa, holding more conversations with Alec Walker. But most newsworthy on this trip was his argument with Dr. Christian Barnard, the South African surgeon who had made headlines doing the first heart transplant.

"Coronary heart disease," Barnard insisted, "is caused by a genetic inability to metabolize some fats, with resultant deposit of cholesterol in the heart's arteries."

"To the contrary," Burkitt declared, standing his ground, "coronary heart disease is entirely preventable and is caused by an improper dietary. I strongly deny a hereditary factor, for Indians in Natal, South Africa have four times more heart attacks than their blood relatives in Southern India. Their heart attacks," he recounted, "are caused by a change in environmental eating habits, not genetic factors."

After Denis returned to his London office, Cleave visited him again. Although Denis freely admitted that Cleave had revolutionized his life and thinking, yet he had great difficulty in talking with him. The captain still held a rigid position on sugar. Having been attacked so often by the medical profession, he refused to accept any criticism or modification of his theory. As a Christian, Denis tried to maintain a good relationship, but it wasn't easy.

Burkitt had always compared any complex medical problem with a jigsaw puzzle. To complete a picture, one needed to fit all the pieces together, exactly. Usually it required many different people working on one disease problem to put together all the pieces and solve the puzzle. In any research project, one had to begin with a hypothesis and endeavor to find evidence to support it. If the evidence failed to agree with a hypothesis, one must modify or abandon it. Those engaged in research couldn't cling to pet ideas and ignore other's valid findings which might not agree with a favored hypothesis. To refuse to put a piece of information in its proper place would be like hiding the key piece of a jigsaw puzzle.

But on September 26, Denis momentarily left all thoughts of medical research as he recorded in his diary a significant Burkitt event: "Philip asked me for Judy's hand in marriage tonight." Judy had finished her training as a teacher and was a

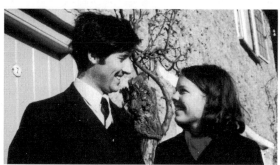

Phillip Howard courts Judy.

gifted educator. Her suitor, Philip Howard, was also a teacher. They confided to Denis and Olive that before considering their own interests, they wanted to give the first two years of their married life in working for the underprivileged. They had decided that teaching orphans in Kenya would fulfill this commitment. Both parents were pleased that Judy wanted to return to Africa.

In October of this demanding year, 1970, Burkitt headed for yet another extensive lecturing and fact-finding trip, this time to include Afghanistan, Pakistan and India, where he planned to visit mission and government hospitals. After returning home in mid-November, he received a letter from the American Leukemia Society stating that he was to receive the Robert de Villiers Award for an "epoch-making discovery in the cause of leukemia." This, he couldn't understand. He sat down immediately, writing a letter remonstrating that he'd never treated a case of leukemia in his life, and surely shouldn't receive the award! However, by return mail came the assurance that he was indeed deserving of the prize because of his contributions to chemotherapy for the related Burkitt's lymphoma.

So, on December 5, he flew to San Juan, where the leukemia conference was convening. Being housed in a luxurious hotel, he couldn't resist making some comparisons, *Two nights in this hotel, without breakfast, cost more than I received in research grants for the first eighteen months of my work on the African lymphoma!* In his diary he wrote: "Feel lonely in this wealthy, materialistic society."

His second daughter's suitor met him on his return to The Knoll. This time a young chap, Andrew Boddam-Whetham, headed for a career in medicine, was asking for the hand of Cassy. The thought of soon losing two daughters to marriage made Denis realize how rapidly time was passing.

*****

Political problems were brewing in Uganda. Since the country had become independent in 1962 under Milton Obote as prime minister, there had been gradual changes. Simultaneous with the appointment of Obote, the Kabaka, or chief, of a prominent Ugandan tribe had been given the more or less honorary title of "president." Then, in 1966, Obote had arranged with army officer Idi Amin to execute the Kabaka, but the assassination attempt had been unsuccessful. From then on, Obote had become both increasingly autocratic and unpopular, leading in 1969 to an attempt on his own life.

Now, in 1971, Idi Amin, who had risen to the position of general of the army, staged a successful coup. At first, the Ugandans were pleased with Obote's downfall. However, the principal of a large mission school viewed the situation more realistically, exclaiming, "This is the biggest disaster that has ever happened to Uganda." Amin, an uneducated boxer and a Moslem, had come up through the ranks of the army. It was said that he had been a good sergeant, a poor lieutenant, and a worse general. He was not even a Ugandan, but a Nubian from southern Sudan.

In 1970 Makerere Medical School had reached its academic zenith with a medical board from London giving accreditation. As far back as 1966, the medical school had appointed its first African dean, while simultaneously placing ever increasing numbers of well-qualified African physicians in other responsible positions. When Michael Hutt left Africa in 1970, he had been confident that the pathology professorship was in good hands, following the appointment of his former assistant in the department. Makerere was but one Ugandan institution to undergo great changes after Amin took over the reigns of government.

*****

Still inspired by the Cook Centennial in Africa, Hugh Trowell sent Denis a copy of his book, *Non-Infective Diseases in Africa*. Burkitt read it through with growing interest.

It's amazing, the insights Hugh had in nutrition, he thought, *and to think that for so many years his work has been completely ignored. In fact, years ago, when it came to choosing the professorship in the department of medicine at Makerere, his interest in nutrition was even held against him!*

Although he immediately acknowledged receipt of the book and frequently dropped Hugh a line from various parts of the world, it was many months before Burkitt actually had time to invite him to his office.

One afternoon as Trowell stood his umbrella in a corner of Denis's office, he said, "I apologize for the mildewed, warped book I sent." Sitting down opposite Burkitt, he continued, "It was a survivor from rain and dampness while it sat in an exposed crate on a dock."

"Never mind, Hugh," Denis said, "it's my turn to apologize for not inviting you sooner to discuss your book with me."

"No need to apologize. Since our brief meeting in Kampala and your questioning me about fiber, I've had time to work on the subject. Do you remember the paper you and Neil Painter were working on regarding 'Fiber and Diverticular Disease of the Colon?' " Hugh asked.

"Yes, and Neil asked you to write a letter to the *British Medical Journal*, giving support for the use of bran for various intestinal conditions," Denis finished.

"I'll admit my surprise at the time." Hugh pushed back a lock of white hair from his forehead. "I couldn't understand why you and Neil were coming out so strongly for the therapeutic properties of bran when the idea was considered heresy by most physicians. I didn't think advocating bran would enhance Painter's medical career either."

"Well, you do know that the fiber and diverticular disease article was published this year—and in an early issue of that very journal!" Denis leaned back in his chair.

"True, but since you and Neil had come out with your surgical article in support of fiber, I thought that an article on atherosclerosis and fiber would possibly open up thought on the medical diseases in a similar way." Trowell unconsciously talked loudly, as he had become quite deaf, a result of taking quinine for years in the tropics. "I had several rejections of my article, but each time I went back again and researched further in the medical literature. Actually, this made me find answers to weak areas in my fiber hypothesis," Hugh said.

"I notice, from a copy of the article you sent me, that you've gone beyond suggesting bran as a treatment, and instead you support the idea that fiber-rich foods are essential for health—that these prevent atherosclerosis and other diseases. Incidentally, I've been impressed that your scope of Western diseases goes far beyond that proposed by Cleave." Denis pulled Hugh's disreputable-looking volume from his bookshelf, turned to the front pages, and said, "I see that your book came out in 1960."

"Yes, but it actually sold only a few copies and was never referenced in medical literature outside of Africa," Trowell admitted.

As Denis turned the pages of the book, he again noticed, by the titles and subtitles, that Trowell and Cleave, quite independently, had made the same general observations.

"Hugh," Burkitt said finally, "for several years, I've been collecting dietary data and statistics which show the absence of Western diseases in Third World countries. In addition, I've done bowel transit-times on all classes of society in Britain and Africa." Burkitt looked intently at Trowell. "I'm considering writing a book on diet and Western diseases. I can claim some competence in the area of surgical diseases, but couldn't write with any authority on medical conditions. You've spent years in the internal medicine specialty, and nutrition has always been your great interest. Would you consider co-operating with me on such a project?"

Highly pleased with the invitation, Hugh immediately agreed to the proposal. "Denis, I don't think I ever told you this bit of personal history, but in my last year of medicine in 1929 at St. Thomas's, when I was a house physician, my professor asked me to find a case of coronary heart disease. They needed to discuss the phenomenon among the medical students."

"In 1929—did you find a case?" Denis asked.

"I had great difficulty in locating a single case in the hospital records department!" Hugh smiled at the remembrance. "It was a rare disease then, but because in America they were beginning to talk about it, the professor thought we should all be aware of the condition, that we should learn its characteristic symptoms, just in case we ever saw a patient with the disease! That one experience made a lasting impression, and I've followed the rising incidence of coronary heart disease with great interest ever since."

"In all your years in Africa, did you ever see a single case, Hugh?"

"Yes, I attended the very first case of coronary heart disease seen in East Africa. The patient was a high court African judge who'd trained in England. He'd obviously changed his dietary habits while in England and retained them after returning to Africa," Trowell recalled. "I felt then that the English diet was certainly a causal factor in his disease."

Denis, thinking ahead, said, "Changing the subject a bit, we'll give Peter Cleave credit for all his work and the findings he's uncovered. In fact, I'd like to dedicate our book to him."

Watching Trowell leave his office that day, Burkitt couldn't help admiring this 65-year-old physician who, perhaps at last, would reap some reward for his years of diligence and keen observation. *And to think Providence brought all of these contacts —Cleave, Walker, Trowell, Dimmock—into my life in perfect order!*

Now, ever more convinced that the Lord was calling him to a wider, more important commitment in medicine, he determined to step even more wholeheartedly into popularizing, not only the neglected field of nutrition, but preventive medicine as well.

15

MORAL FIBER

The longer Denis worked on the Western dietary problem, the more convinced he became that his best contribution to medicine might become, not to cure, but to prevent, some of the world's most serious diseases. As he viewed certain illnesses now termed "Western diseases," he observed that few of them had been present to any extent fifty years earlier.

In 1971, coronary heart disease had become the commonest cause of death in the Western world; appendicitis, the most frequent emergency surgical operation; gallstones, the most often-repeated elective surgical procedure; diverticular disease of the colon, the most prevalent lesion in the large bowel; obesity, a 20th century "epidemic" in the West; diabetes, the predominant metabolic disorder; cancer of the colon, the second most common cancer in men and third in women; hemorrhoids and varicose veins, relatively new "plagues"; and hiatus hernia, a unique affliction, exclusive to the West.

In gathering dietary information from his Third World contacts, certain facts were becoming obvious. Unrefined, simple foods were the most common nutrients in all these nations. They used rice, corn, wheat, millet, barley and potatoes (mostly yams), as well as various legumes—soybeans, red beans and lentils—according to their cultures. These were the staples. Because of poverty, there were few dairy products, eggs or red meat. They ate fish more commonly than meat, but even so, rarely. The use of tuber vegetables or leafy plants varied considerably from country to country. Fruits of all kinds in the diet depended entirely upon their availability and cost in a given country.

Quite obviously, these diets, mostly consisting of unrefined carbohydrates, were rich in fiber which, in turn, absorbed water from the bowel, producing large, soft stools. At the same time, their food was low in fat. Denis had agreed that fat should be eaten sparingly.

As he studied Hugh Trowell's 1960 book, *Non-Infective Disease in Africa*, Denis noticed that Hugh had a comprehensive list of over thirty Western diseases. The 480-page book reflected the thoroughness with which he studied a subject, for it had over 1,700 references. Trowell had drawn attention to the Africans' starchy food, rich in "roughage," producing soft bulky stools, and he had suggested that it provided protection, particularly against gastrointestinal disease. During their visits, Denis admired this man more than ever for his insight and pioneer work. *What a pity this book has passed unnoticed by the Western medical press!* Denis thought. Trowell gave "dietary fiber" its name, as well as its definition as "that part of plant food which is undigested by the enzymes of the human digestive tract."

Burkitt introduced Trowell to Cleave, and they had met on several occasions. Hugh found Cleave quite unbending in his ideas and he, like Denis, made no progress in getting Cleave to acknowledge the part that fat played in Western diseases, although Cleave did admit to fiber's minor role. Denis realized, from his lymphoma experience, that one has to be willing to admit errors and modify ideas. Nevertheless, he had great regard for Cleave, even though the captain often became upset if Denis departed at all from his own original ideas. Cleave's hypothesis was not open to modification. It was the gospel in his eyes!

All the time Denis and Trowell worked together, Hugh was suffering from a severe handicap. He came to liken himself to St. Paul in prison writing letters from his dungeon cell. Because of his deafness, Hugh spent hours in libraries. Later, he was "imprisoned" not only his by deafness but also by his beloved wife's disability, for he tended her himself.

Simultaneously, while Denis was working with Trowell, he was writing a paper with his old Scot friend from house-surgeon-training days, Conrad Latto. Latto, now a senior surgical consultant at the Royal Berkshire Hospital in Reading, had also become interested in the attributes of fiber. Conrad's interest in fiber was compounded since he himself had been a lifelong vegetarian. At his Reading hospital, Latto had studied one hundred patients with diverticular disease and had found that the majority of them also had varicose veins. These two Western diseases, appearing together, were to him and Denis a demonstration of a "common cause" worthy of a medical report.

After talking with Cleave and Burkitt, Latto introduced a revolutionary regime into his surgical ward. Each morning his patients were given a medicine-cup-full of bran on their porridge. This highly successful experiment led to the abandonment of laxatives for his postoperative patients. The practice actually started a "bran wave" in the community. When the patients went home, they continued using bran and encouraged its use among their neighbors.

Initially, other surgeons in the hospital considered the bran treatment as quackery. Even Latto's chief resident was skeptical, thinking the whole project "rubbish." Conrad, however, wanting to prove his point, suggested, "Why don't the two of us run a test? I'll take the bran, but both of us will ingest two capsules of carmine dye. Then we'll determine our bowel transit-times."

"But I'm not constipated!" the resident physician objected.

"We'll see," his chief said.

Both swallowed the capsules, and Conrad the bran in addition. Within twenty-four hours, the carmine dye appeared in Latto's stools. Six days later the dye showed in the resident's stools. Needless to say, the younger man also became a bran-advocate.

*****

In February 1971, when Denis planned a safari through a primitive part of East Africa and Malawi, he invited his good friends Ralph and Ruth Blocksma to accompany him. Since Ralph always tithed his time, committing six weeks a year to some active mission service, he responded enthusiastically to the suggestion. The three of them left from London, sitting together in a row on their flight to Entebbe.

"When you finish using your salt and pepper, save them for me," Denis requested. "Also, if you don't use your plastic packets of jam and peanut butter, I'll take those too."

Ralph looked at him with some surprise, but complied with the request. Half jokingly, he asked, "Anything else you want, Denis?"

"Yes, let's keep our plastic dinnerware. You'll see that these will come in handy," Denis promised as he tucked some of the items in his air-flight bag.

After landing in Entebbe, they found the townspeople in a mood of rejoicing, having planted the roadsides with young banana trees in celebration of the bloodless coup recently accomplished by Idi Amin.

"Ever since independence, there's been increasing political unrest in Uganda," Denis observed. "We can only hope there'll soon be peaceful solutions to the country's many problems."

After a brief stop in Kampala to renew friendships and check on the progress of the Burkitt lymphoma studies, they flew on to Lilongwe, the capital of Malawi. Here, Denis rented a small European sedan, "a good car, so Ruth can be comfortable." Each day as they traveled through previously unvisited areas of Malawi, they stopped at two or more mission hospitals.

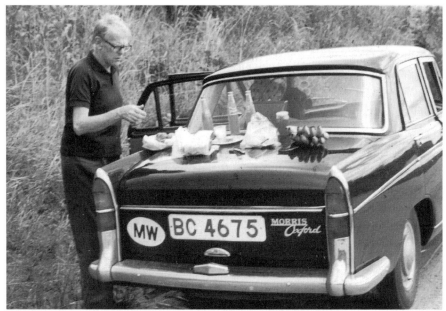

Time out for a picnic lunch on the Malawi safari.

After several days had passed, Ralph cautiously asked, "Denis, how is it that we always seem to arrive at a hospital at mealtime? It's a bit embarrassing."

"I'm sure people are delighted to see us. We'll be arriving at the next hospital just before lunch," Denis advised, as he stepped a little more firmly on the throttle. True to his word, they pulled into the grounds of a hospital just as the doctor's family was sitting down to eat.

"Say, have you folks eaten yet?" the doctor asked.

"Matter of fact, we haven't," Denis said, flashing his winsome smile. And they were soon seated at the dining table. Many times, of course, they would be out on a lonely stretch of road when it was time to eat. But Denis was prepared. He made a habit of stopping to buy a few things in a local bazaar. Then, spreading the food out on the trunk of the car, he would produce the extras saved from their airline trays, including the plastic dinnerware. It was little wonder his safari expense accounts were so small!

In addition, he sought out inexpensive accommodations for the night. One especially memorable rest house Denis nicknamed the Kota-Kota Hilton. It was a dilapidated affair decorated with old car parts—fenders and bumpers around the eves, and car doors with wind-down windows serving that same purpose in the crude building. The linens on the beds were dirty, and bats slept by day in the rafters. In the morning when they were eating breakfast, they found that the roof leaked torrents of rain.

As their journey continued, Denis felt he'd seldom met anyone quite like Ralph, who so constantly sought opportunities to give. Blocksma had brought along surgical instruments to perform any plastic surgery needed at the various mission hospitals they visited. Part way through the trip, they stopped at a mission hospital where the young doctor, trained in surgery, had little equipment.. Ralph promptly unrolled his carefully packed fine instruments and commented, "God has been very good to me. I would like you to have these."

This is Ralph Blocksma, Denis thought, *always so generous!*

At each hospital, Burkitt meticulously gathered his data, patiently and respectfully probing for information from each doctor, many of them black. He inquired not only about the diseases which the doctors saw, but those which they never encountered. He visited the kitchens and observed exactly what fare the patients ate. Most of the time this proved to be huge mounds of yams and brown rice—fiber-rich food. Denis repeatedly showed Ralph and Ruth that their diets consisted entirely of unrefined carbohydrate.

"They rarely eat any meat and consequently their diet is relatively low in protein and very low in fat. Yet," Denis continued, "most of the people in these areas have good general health, not counting their parasites and infections." This was an education for the Blocksmas. They could certainly see the difference in the pattern

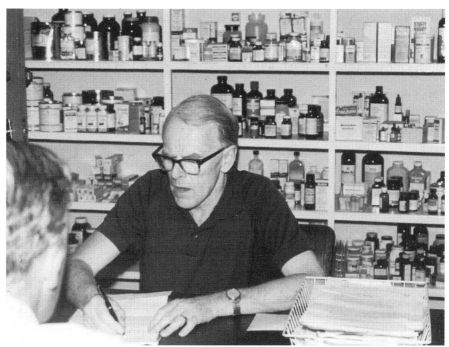

Burkitt queries a doctor regarding diet and disease in Malawi.

185

of diseases from that of the Western world. On the safari, they hadn't seen a single patient with a Western disease.

Some of the time Denis followed the same route David Livingston had taken many years before. However, February was not proving to be the best time of year for the trip with its occasional torrential rains making the unpaved roads seas of mud. More than once, the little car became immobile in a morass up to the bumpers. On one occasion, they became impossibly stuck in the middle of nowhere. Suddenly, unexpectedly, a swarm of black "angels" appeared, who bodily lifted the car out of the muck onto firmer soft clay.

As they drove one day through a completely deserted area of Malawi in their "comfortable sedan," the car chose this spot to overheat. Although Denis didn't profess to know much about auto mechanics, he lifted the hot hood of the mud-encrusted car. With a cursory examination, he came up with the diagnosis, a loose fan belt. He quickly adjusted the tension, so that the worn belt functioned again. With this trouble attended to, they made it to a rest house. There, another traveler in a Land Rover had an array of fan belts in his tool case, one an exact fit for their car. "You can't say the Lord doesn't take care of His own!" Denis wiped his greasy hands on a rag after he'd finished installing the new belt.

As they were completing their Malawi safari, they came upon a perfect dental demonstration of the Western dietary effect. An elderly African who'd cooked for a European family had, quite obviously, enjoyed some of his rich culinary products

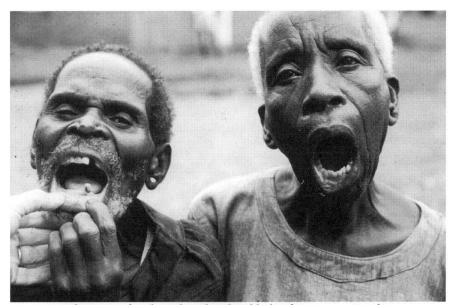

Left: Foreign family cook and Right: elderly African on native diet.
They are comparing teeth.

for years. Ralph took a picture of him and another nearby African patriarch. The cook's nearly toothless lower jaw compared poorly with the perfect teeth of the other white-haired African, who had eaten only the native diet throughout his life.

During this particular African trip, after the Blocksmas had left him, Denis visited briefly with Dr. Ted Williams. Ted had kept excellent records since their historic long safari ten years previously. He now had a sizable tumor registry, albeit in a grass-thatched mud hut.

Since his hospital was "in the bush," Ted had developed his own routine for children suspected of having BL. He treated each of the patients as an emergency, for indeed, they were, as the tumor always progressed rapidly. He would immediately take the child to the surgery and under anesthetic, take a biopsy of the tumor. With the child still asleep, he would touch the cut surface of the tumor to a clean microscopic slide, stain the "touch preparation," and read the slide himself under a microscope. Ted had become proficient under Hutt's and Wright's tutelage in diagnosing the tumor from the stained cell preparation.

After making a diagnosis of BL, he would immediately inject a chemotherapeutic agent into the child's peritoneal cavity, repeating the injection on the third day. Ted had an excellent record of survivors who experienced rapid and permanent regression of the tumor. The diagnosis was always later confirmed with the biopsy sent to Mulago. Through his careful work, Williams would continue to make valuable contributions by publishing additional scientific papers on different aspects of the disease.

*****

April 1971 saw Denis in Lyon, France at the International Agency for Research in Cancer. Since he had researched esophageal carcinoma as one of the seven cancers in his African geographical studies, Burkitt related his experience with the disease at the conference. While in Lyon, he met Dr. Guy de-The', who was working with this cancer agency and spoke with him regarding Ted Williams' investigation of BL in Uganda. Dr. de-The' would later work with Williams at the Kuluva Hospital on a massive lymphoma project.

Even though Burkitt had been doing bowel transit-times for years, he noticed a hiatus in his research, the bowel habits of vegetarians. He expected to find very different bowel transit-times in vegetarians from those he'd been observing in meat-eaters. Vegetarians, eating a diet high in plant fiber, eliminate high-calorie meat, which is completely devoid of fiber. Knowing that Seventh-day Adventists (SDAs) are largely vegetarians, he arranged to do studies at their St. Christopher's school in England. There, he did bowel transit times on a large segment of the student body. These students *did have* reduced transit-times when compared with other English school children.

Later that year, when in California, he visited the Seventh-day Adventist medical school in Loma Linda, where he gathered further data on vegetarians. He found supporting statistics from the report of Doctors Ernest Wynder and Frank Lemon, who had compared the occurrence of several diseases between California SDAs and a segment of other Californians. They found that the largely vegetarian SDAs had only fifty-nine percent of cancer deaths suffered by meat-eaters; fifty-five percent of coronary heart disease deaths; fifty-five percent diabetic deaths; and fifty-three percent of deaths from strokes. These statistics supported the thesis that a fiber-rich diet provides a high degree of protection from Western diseases.

On this same United States trip, he visited the Mormon medical school at Brigham Young University in Salt Lake City, Utah. Mormon statistics also revealed a lower rate of coronary heart disease, bowel cancer and diabetes. He learned that many Mormons grind their own wheat, from which they bake whole grain bread. However, Mormons are beef-eaters. Denis postulated that perhaps their increased dietary fiber protected them from the atherogenic, saturated fat in the meat.

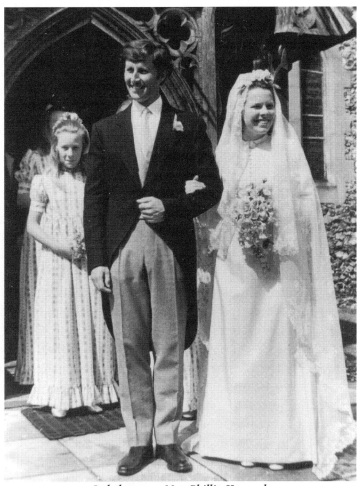

Judy becomes Mrs. Phillip Howard.

*****

188

Without a doubt the highlight of 1971 was the marriage of Judy to Philip Howard on July 24. Denis himself had mowed and trimmed the grounds of The Knoll to perfection, for the spacious yard lent itself well to the reception of the wedding guests. As a precaution, they had a large canvas awning erected for protective seating in case of rain. This family celebration gave Denis a first opportunity to don his fine morning suit, purchased secondhand years before.

The wedding proved a brief but pleasant interlude in his busy schedule. In September, Denis had an interview with a woman administrator of the British Nutrition Foundation (BNF), which, he soon learned, was financially-supported and dominated by the food industry. He discussed his and Trowell's fiber research with the interested lady administrator, who suggested he write a paper on the subject and submit it to the Foundation for publication. This he did without delay. She promptly replied, saying that the "excellent article" had been received. A few days later, however, she phoned to tell Burkitt that the "authorities" wouldn't allow its publication.

Denis had recently spent time with Professor Sir Ernst Chain, the synthesizer of penicillin, who had told him of his own previous interest in fiber. Now, as Denis put down the phone after talking with the administrator of the BNF, the phone rang again. This time it was Sir Ernst Chain on the line. Denis mentioned his disappointment at having his fiber article rejected after he'd been asked to write it.

Chain laughed, "I'm not too surprised. You know that the millers are powerful and pretty much control what is published by the BNF. But I happen to be on their board of scientific advisers, and I'll see what I can do."

A few days later Denis received a message from the British Nutrition Foundation advising him that they were pleased to publish his paper. Sir Ernst repeatedly proved a great moral support to Burkitt and Trowell as they pursued their research and writing.

*****

Denis had become increasingly in demand as a speaker at various medical functions. The medical profession, at least, was beginning to listen to the message which he, Cleave, Walker and Trowell were espousing. In October, Denis traveled to his native Ireland for a nutritional conference held at the National University in Dublin. There he learned an interesting tidbit from Dr. James Fennelly, who had been investigating the diet of the Irish. Before the Irish potato famine in the middle of the nineteenth century, Irish laborers had lived on a pint of milk and ten pounds of potatoes a day.

Amazing, thought Denis, *that such a simple diet could support healthy, strong working men. Obviously, we have been overlooking the benefits of many nutri-*

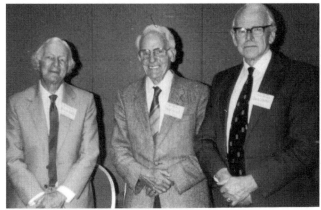

Left to right: Alec Walker, Hugh Trowell and Denis Burkitt, pioneers in finding causes of Western diseases.

tious foods for years. He learned that the potato was a good source of fiber, although it contains less fiber, weight-for-weight, than bread. The potato is 90% water, whereas whole-grain bread is about 33% water.

Not only the medical profession, but also the public was beginning to hear about fiber. Before leaving for meetings in Iran and an extensive lecture and fact-finding trip through India, Denis was interviewed for a television program, "Men and Ideas." He made the most of television or radio opportunities to lay facts of proper nutrition before the public, emphasizing the benefits of unrefined foods and fiber. The British people were slowly awakening, but not fast enough to suit Denis and Hugh.

At the close of 1971, after finishing an article on varicose veins, he counted twelve published articles for the year. His nutritional research had recorded changes in disease patterns in Japan, Malaysia, New Zealand and Canadian Eskimos with their emerging Western diseases. He had noted the high incidence of diabetes among the Pima Indians in Southwestern United States. Looking over his diary for the year, he also recalled five international trips, not counting those to Scotland and Ireland. He had lectured on every continent, condemning present milling processes with high bran extraction.

During these lectures, he had developed a motto: "The browner, the better; the whiter, the worse. 'B' for brown and better; 'W' for white and worse!" Then he had described fiber's role from the mouth to the rectum, covering the entire gamut of Western diseases. He had loudly emphasized that the widely diverse array of the Western world's plague diseases was preventable. Gradually, the public, especially in the United States, thanks to wide exposure by the media, was beginning to respond.

But not without a struggle. There were vested interests to convince as well!

16

WALKING THE SECOND MILE

When FIBER burst upon TV screens, radio waves, billboards, and magazine advertisements and festooned every box of dry cereal flakes, FIBER became the "in" word. Food companies proclaimed it as nearly a magical "cure-all." Of course, fiber was but one of several dietary factors nutritional researchers began emphasizing simultaneously. The new message was: reduce saturated fat, use complex carbohydrates (plant foods, rich in fiber), watch the salt (actually the sodium), reduce the sugar, and lower the animal proteins.

"Authorities" suddenly appeared, stating that FIBER was the only generally common food component *deficient* in the Western diet. This claim gave fiber-depleted diets a considerable responsibility for the ravages of the so-called Western diseases. At last FIBER had come into its own as an important part of the diet.

However, in 1972, FIBER'S time had *not yet come* in Britain. Although the United States was beginning to play the scenario, in Britain it was still a hoped-for dream in the minds of a few earnest investigators. Indeed, the success that FIBER would later enjoy in Britain did not come without a *long* struggle.

There were still misunderstandings between even Cleave and the collaborators, Burkitt and Trowell. When the three met, Denis again tried to point out the importance of fiber-depleted diets above excessive sugar as paramount in causing Western diseases.

"As you know, Peter," he reminded Cleave, when he once more opened the controversial subject, "for the past several years I've been collecting data from a thousand mission hospitals around the world besides personally going on fact-finding safaris to Africa, Asia, and North and South America. I've conducted and compared countless bowel transit-time stool studies in the Western and Third Worlds. As a result, both Trowell and I firmly believe that fiber-deficiency can be identified as a missing, important factor in the Western diet and that it plays an enormously important role in causing Western diseases, even diabetes."

"I know. You've stressed this before, Denis, many times," said Cleave.

"I've spent endless hours in researching medical literature on the subject of fiber," Hugh added, "and we're not alone in suspecting that a fiber-deficient diet causes many bowel disorders."

"All right, but I'd like to point out some statistics from both World Wars," Cleave declared. "During the wars, there was a sugar shortage, and diabetic deaths fell during 1914–18 and again in 1941–48."

Denis agreed, but suggested, "Let's look at another principle factor of the wartime diet." He was using facts accrued by Trowell. "You'll remember, Peter, that the government requested the millers to extract less bran from the wheat so as to produce more flour. Instead of the fiber-depleted white bread which the people had previously eaten, during the war all were eating the 'National Loaf,' an eighty-five percent whole wheat bread."

Hugh added the clincher. "When sugar consumption went back to prewar levels in 1953, the diabetes incidence didn't rise. This was because the high-fiber National Loaf was still the staple, and remained so until 1954. It wasn't until after the bakers reintroduced white bread that diabetes flourished again, in 1956."

Cleave changed the subject saying, "Denis, you're always talking about fiber preventing diverticulosis. But sugar is the real problem there too."

Denis hesitated to add further fuel to the fire but said with a sigh, "Peter, don't you think that sugar is pretty well absorbed by the time the food reaches the colon, and especially the sigmoid colon, where we find most of the diverticula?"

Even these bits of evidence didn't sway Cleave as he clung to his saccharine theory as the cause of Western diseases and of diabetes in particular. This confrontation, unfortunately, was by no means the end of the controversy.

Conrad Latto met Cleave at the McCarrison Society, both being members of this organization. A group of doctors and dentists who promoted health and prevention of disease through sound nutrition had founded the society in 1966. They'd named it after Sir Robert McCarrison, a famous nutritional scientist, who, in the early 1900's, warned against processing and refining. McCarrison had promoted minimally-processed foods. Conrad got on well with Cleave and proved to be a mediator when there was disagreement over the varicose vein paper which Denis was writing and had sent to Cleave for comment.

Thus, on February 15, 1972, Denis wrote two bits of news in his diary: "Critical letter from Cleave disagreeing with varicose vein paper. Academic Press gladly accepted the proposal for our book." This was the book he and Trowell were working on. A few days later, he received a phone call from Conrad.

"I do believe that Cleave is allergic to you, Denis," Conrad said, stifling a laugh. "I would advise that you simply remain silent when he expounds on his theory. It only irritates him when you offer a counter idea."

"How true! Thanks for your advice, Conrad," Denis said. "You know I really love the man. I admire him. And besides, I owe him a great debt for opening my eyes to this whole nutrition problem. But he's one man I haven't learned how to deal with. I'll sit right down and write an apology for my part in the disagreement."

Denis immediately followed through on his intention. The following day he received a phone call from Cleave saying that his letter, just received, totally altered the situation. Within a couple of weeks, Conrad called again to say he thought Cleave had accepted Denis's suggested changes in the varicose vein paper.

In spite of his various commitments, Burkitt never allowed scientific matters to crowd out association with other Christians. At the end of January, Olive and he had hosted a Christian Medical Fellowship party in their home for medical students. Denis enjoyed keeping in touch with the younger generation of would-be physicians, often trying to inspire them with the need for more preventive measures in medical care. On this occasion, one of the medical students he and Olive met was David Maurice, never imagining that he would one day become the husband of their youngest daughter, Rachel.

As March drew on, Denis was in a quandary. He was to receive a gold medal for his work on the lymphoma from the Society of Apothecaries in London. It was a most formal affair to which he must wear a white tie and tails. But he had no such suit and was reluctant to buy one for a single occasion. In voicing his predicament to a friend in his village, the man surprised him by saying he had tails and no use for them. He'd been about to give them to a jumble sale. Bringing Denis the suit, he suggested that he try it on, which he did.

"A perfect fit! It's yours," the neighbor exclaimed.

"If only all my problems could be solved that easily!" Denis said, giving a hearty thanks to his friend.

Within a week, Denis again wrote in his diary, March 5: "It distresses me that Peter Cleave and I have not been able to come to agreement. He does not reciprocate my apologies. This is an opportunity as a Christian to try to show love and give help. Conrad is so helpful." On March 7, he wrote: "Gold medal from Society of Apothecaries. Got varicose vein paper back with more requests for additions by Cleave. This upset me. Worried about his disagreement. Must get over this."

Mid-March found Denis, Olive and Cassy traveling by ship across the English channel to two appointments on the Continent. After disembarking, they caught a train to Heidelberg, where he lectured prior to their traveling on to Frankfurt for his receipt of the Paul Ehrlich-Ludwig Darmstaedter gold medal. For Cassy the trip was an exciting interlude between her just-completed physiotherapy training and her wedding. She had never before had an opportunity to attend an affair where her father was honored for his contributions to medical progress.

As they rested in their luxurious hotel rooms awaiting the event, all three were impressed with German hospitality. They were regaled with beautiful flower arrangements and trolleys of fresh fruit. But match folders imprinted with "D.P. Burkitt," were the most unusual mementos. The Germans had forgotten nothing!

The presentation of the medal proved a newsworthy occasion with high government dignitaries as well as eminent scientists in attendance. Denis ended his acceptance speech with a particularly poignant remark, "I only wish my mother could have been present on this occasion." He never failed to remember how much his dear mother had contributed to his life's success.

Leaving Olive and Cassy in Frankfurt, he flew directly to New York for another hectic tour. By this time, most of his lectures were on fiber and the Western diseases. Fortunately, American audiences were ready and eager to consider what Burkitt had to say.

At the Buttersworth Hospital in Grand Rapids, he suffered embarrassment when the medical staff rose with a standing ovation after his lecture. However, across town in another hospital, devoted largely to gastrointestinal diseases, he met with criticism behind his back. After his lecture emphasizing the new dietary slant on preventing many gastrointestinal diseases, the chief surgeon came up to Ralph Blocksma, who had introduced Burkitt to the staff and commented, "Ralph, this guy Burkitt is a quack."

Ralph understood the exact reason for the disparaging statement. Following Burkitt's advice would put a lot of surgeons nearly out of business. On their way home, he told Denis about the remark.

"Never mind," Denis said. "I spent twenty years 'mopping up' until I learned it was wiser to 'turn off the tap.' " He was referring to a favorite cartoon used in his lectures that depicted doctors mopping the floor while water still spilled from an overflowing basin under an opened faucet. His point was that prevention of many diseases, "turning off the tap," could easily prevent the "mopping up" therapeutic and surgical procedures carried out by most physicians.

While Denis was visiting the Blocksmas in Grand Rapids, Michigan, Ralph took him to the Kellogg Company in nearby Battle Creek. Denis talked to the executive staff at the plant, who received him cordially, but he got the feeling that they considered themselves already knowledgeable on fiber. After all, hadn't they been manufacturing All Bran for scores of years? This was old stuff to them.

However, he was to find that circumstances would change—rapidly. No sooner did he return to his London office, than he received a phone call from Kellogg's inquiring the date of his next American tour. If he would let them know the time of his arrival in New York, they would send a private executive jet to meet him. They wanted their regional representatives to gather so that he could talk to them. This meeting was to prove the beginning of a supportive relationship with the Kellogg Company. However, he was careful never to promote their products or those of any other food company.

After the initial visit to Kellogg's, while still on his U.S. tour, he was struck one morning by his devotional reading of Matthew 26:30–35. In this text, the apostle Peter had been self-confident that he would never forsake Jesus in the coming crisis before the Lord's crucifixion. As Denis thought about this Bible scene, he wrote in his diary: "We are all liable to fall away from our faith. Human will, determination and dedication are insufficient. It requires His Spirit in us to hold us. Jesus prepared for His greatest test by praying alone. This is our best preparation, not only for crises, but for each day." His diary entry that day reflected Burkitt's determination to remain a simple, devoted Christian, regardless of what controversy or honor might come to him.

His next stop was Chicago, where he lectured mission doctors who had gathered for an M.A.P. convention. Denis often marveled at how his various speaking invitations dovetailed conveniently. However, he made it a practice to notify local Christian Medical Societies of the dates when he would be in an area at the expense of another medical society. In this way, he could fellowship with his Christian friends and they, in turn, could profit by his visits without monetary outlay.

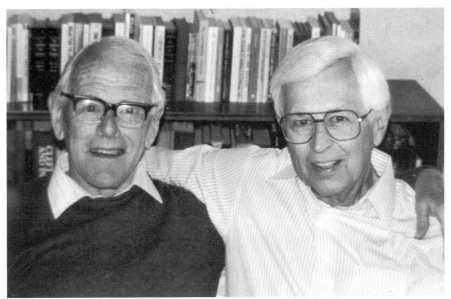

Old friends, Denis Burkitt and Ralph Blocksma

Yet another honor awaited him on his arrival home. He would become a fellow of the Royal Society in April. *How is it*, he wondered, *that I am to receive this top accolade given to scientists in this country? I don't suppose more than one physician a year is elected to this select body. I'm in no sense a "scientist,"* he thought, apologetically. *However, this fellowship will give me added credibility and will certainly be an asset in giving acceptance to the nutritional gospel I'm promoting.*

*****

April 8th, 1972 was the big day for Cassy and Andrew. Once again the grounds preparation at the Knoll for the wedding occupied the family. It was Andrew's and Cassy's plan, shortly after their marriage, to go as medical missionaries to Kenya. Africa would soon claim two Burkitt daughters, both Judy and Cassy.

With the wedding only a month behind, on May 9, Denis gave the Walker prize lecture for the Royal College of Surgeons. The number of coveted prizes he was receiving for his work on the lymphoma overwhelmed him. "I'm so unworthy!" he kept remonstrating. His favorite text for this, 1 Corinthians 4:7, said it all: "What have you got that you did not receive, and if you received it all as a gift, why take the credit to yourself?"

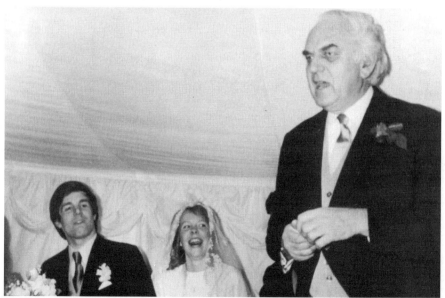

*Doctor Conrad Latto offers humorous advice at Andrew and
Cassy's wedding reception.*

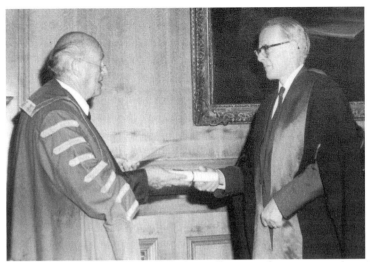

Burkitt receives the Walker award.

Also in May 1972, the Radiology Society in London invited him to give a memorial lecture. Even before his presentation, the *British Medical Journal* asked if they could publish the text. This was an unusual request. A friend had previously warned Denis that many researchers considered scientifically unsound the idea that a single factor (such as a fiber-depleted diet) could cause many diseases. Such an article promoting this concept, he'd been told, had little likelihood of being accepted for publication. However, before the journal editors knew the topic of his lecture, they had accepted his manuscript, simply because it was written by Denis Burkitt, the physician who was being recognized and honored worldwide for his scientific accomplishments.

Burkitt then presented his well-attended lecture entitled, "Some Diseases Characteristic of Modern Western Civilization." In it, he suggested a high-fiber diet might be protective against *all* of these diseases. This concept, relatively new at the time, caught on immediately and resulted in newspaper and radio interviews on the subject. But there were critics of the fiber proposal. Since the *British Medical Journal* had previously requested the lecture, its editors were now obligated to print the controversial article. *How providential that they actually requested it first!* Denis observed.

A few days later, while on holiday with Olive in Scotland, he read a press release from the British millers dated May 18, 1972, with growing indignation:

> It is postulated that [certain] diseases are more common in Western countries because of the much greater consumption of refined carbohydrate in the form of white bread and white sugar which, it is claimed, results in a diet of a low fiber, or low residue, content.

"Can you even guess who the millers are referring to in this press release?" Denis called excitedly to Olive as he read the opening paragraph. "They must have been listening to the radio or reading their newspapers about the lecture I just gave in London. Let's see what else they have to say. It's a rather long article."

> The flour milling industry has been advised for many years, and continues to be so advised, by the most eminent medical and scientific authorities available. Its advisers have reached the view that there is no convincing experimental or direct evidence to justify the existence of any link between diverticulosis and these other non-infective diseases of the bowel, and diet in general, much less a link with individual items of our diet.

"I'd really like to know who their 'medical and scientific authorities' are," Denis muttered. "I'll write or contact them when we get back home." He continued to read more of the release.

> Much of the background evidence which has been advanced is regarded as selective, and many cogent factors appear to have been ignored. In the context in question, comparison between the U.K. and primitive communities is not considered to be meaningful.... Life expectancy is not comparable (members of these primitive communities do not normally survive to the age level at which the middle age complaints of our society occur), nor does the degree of medical facilities and medical supervision, on which meaningful observations can be based, permit direct and reliable comparison as between the two communities.

"What do they know about Africa?" Denis exclaimed, chuckling. "They have the same misconception many have about the life-expectancy of the Africans. The African low average life-expectancy is because of high infant mortality, not because the Africans don't live to advanced ages! And many of the newer medical facilities in Africa, like our new Mulago Hospital, rival those in the U.K. What's their next point?"

> The suggestion that there is one single simple explanation to so many different and complex types of disease at once renders it suspect.

"There it is!" he exclaimed, "exactly as my friend warned me. To promote a 'single cause' for the Western diseases would seem quite illogical to most people, let alone doctors." Denis read on.

> As said already, there is no single piece of convincing experimental evidence to support this and in fact evidence from such records as are available of our national diet suggests that the fiber content of the diet today is no lower—and indeed tends to be higher—than at any time during the present century.

"I fear they are forgetting the eras of the World Wars," Denis said. "Even the millers cooperated during the wars in producing flour with a high bran content!" Excitedly, he continued.

> In relation to the reported increasing incidence of diseases of the colon, much significance appears to have been attached to the supposition that white bread, free of fiber, was newly introduced largely as a result of the roller milling of flour towards the end of the last century. This is a complete misconception. There is considerable historical evidence that white bread, in spite of its price, had been accepted as the bread of the ordinary people. And by 1865 the white loaf had already become cheaper than the brown.

"Is that true, Denis? Olive asked. "I always thought that only the royalty and wealthy ate white bread in the last century. They were the ones that were obese and had gout. I thought that the common people ate simple, unrefined food, largely because that's all they could afford."

"It's true, the steel rolling mills did produce cheap refined white flour. Hugh was really concerned about this, he told me." Denis drew a quick breath. "He said he'd researched this point. If the people began eating white bread as a staple back in the late 1800's, he wondered why the Western diseases hadn't occurred earlier—if our fiber theory were to hold true."

"What's the answer?" Olive was caught up in this new fiber mystery.

"Leave it to Hugh's thorough researching! He found that bread consumption had actually fallen at this time."

"Really? Why?" Olive too was learning a bit of history.

"Potatoes had been introduced from America, and by then were being widely cultivated and eaten. Potatoes were cheaper than bread. They had good fiber too. Remember when I came home from Dublin last year and told you about the diet of the Irish laborers before the potato famine? They ate ten pounds of potatoes and a pint of milk a day." Denis turned back to the press release and continued to read.

> Against this background the industry affirms that in its view there is no evidence revealing any significant difference, in relation to health, between present day white bread and whole-meal bread, both of which are extremely good and nutritious foods. Whether eaten as white or whole meal, bread is our most important staple food and as Professor McCance, lately Professor of Experimental Medicine at Cambridge, has pointed out: "Discussions on the relative merits of white and whole-meal bread are usually directed more by psychological bias than by experimental facts."

"Do you know Professor McCance?" Olive asked. "Perhaps he's one of the 'authorities' they're quoting." She marveled at the confidence her husband still maintained in view of this outburst of criticism by the millers.

"I'm surprised at his statement," Denis said. "McCance is a well-known food analyst and a colleague of Hugh's, who's supplied him with information on wartime diets. He wanted Hugh to call fiber 'unavailable carbohydrate.' But this term sounded like fiber was useless to the body, so Hugh wouldn't use it. It's true, Trowell and McCance haven't always seen eye to eye."

"It sounds as though there will be a few tough battles in the near future," Olive forecast.

Denis rubbed his jaw as he contemplated what his next move should be. "If the millers made this kind of a press release, they should be morally bound to say who their 'eminent authorities' are." He sat down that very day and wrote a letter to the originator of the press release, asking the names of the scientists to whom they had referred, so that he might contact them. He added that current work might indicate they had been misled in their conclusions.

Upon returning home from Scotland, Denis had a letter waiting from the millers, which said that they were unable to name their consulting scientists. With this unexpected response, Denis next wrote for an invitation to meet some of the senior milling officials to discuss the matter. They agreed to his proposal.

A series of discussions between Burkitt and Trowell and executives of the British milling industry resulted. Denis was sympathetic with the millers, realizing they had spent the past hundred years using every possible expertise trying to get more and more fiber out of their flour in making whiter and whiter bread. As they saw it, they were producing a purer and purer product. They had, of course, felt threatened by Denis' lecture, listing diseases resulting from a fiber-deficient, highly refined diet.

Initially, the millers felt the idea quite ridiculous, that fiber was nutritionally valuable. They'd been given assurance by the best scientists in England to back up their statements. When Burkitt and Trowell met with them, there was no mutual agreement. But the two physicians went out of their way to keep a discussion going on a friendly basis, even with total disagreement. Neither side attacked the other. The meetings continued periodically for over a year.

As a result of the friendly dialogue, the officials actually invited Burkitt to address the annual meeting of the British millers. A friend laughingly told Burkitt it would be like the "David and Goliath" incident, and Denis would be "David." Burkitt was careful in preparing the lecture to avoid criticizing. He simply presented the facts, with his usual dose of Irish humor.

Not long afterward, the British Bakers also invited him to address their annual meeting. Next came an invitation to attend and lecture at the annual conference of American Millers. He knew these opportunities had come only because he and Hugh had maintained a friendly relationship with the millers.

A compromise eventually settled the case between Burkitt-Trowell and the millers. They put the whole matter before the Committee on the Medical Aspects of Nutrition (COMA N). *This committee is well-named*, Denis thought, *it will probably take them a long time to reach a decision*. Little did he realize just *how* long the committee would be in their COMA!

*****

Conrad Latto, fully supporting Denis in his dietary convictions, accompanied him on a September 1972 African safari. Never having previously visited this continent, Conrad was thrilled at seeing East, West and South Africa by car and plane. Denis introduced him to all the possible terrain— from the arid desert to the spectacular humid equatorial tropics and the cool mountain highlands.

During the trip, Conrad was amazed as he watched his old friend extract information here and there with a bit of "blarney" thrown in. Only now, as he saw the human dynamo at the work he dearly loved, could he appreciate the tremendous expenditure of time and energy represented in each of Denis's lectures and medical articles.

As a result of his exposure to the vast medical needs of Africa, Latto initiated a six-month rotation for his surgical residents in England. He arranged that they take leave from Reading and spend time in the large, new, interdenominational hospital at Moshi in Tanzania. Their training was to include emergency flights with the Flying Doctor Service. This plan was such a success, that his residents, who thoroughly enjoyed the excitement and unusual surgical experiences, hated to return to the humdrum of medical practice in England.

*****

Yet another award came for Denis in November 1972. He flew the Atlantic, first lecturing in New York, Cleveland, Wichita, and Toronto with several radio interviews included. Olive joined him in New York, where he received the Albert Lasker Award. Accommodated there in a "frightfully prestigious" hotel, Denis considered the courtesy "enormously extravagant and unnecessary."

While housed under these circumstances, his Bible reading of 1 John 3 gave him food for thought, which he expressed in his diary: "Christ came to change men's attitudes to God, to neighbor, to money, to sex, to work, to all life. He wasn't much interested in ability, achievement, attainment, acquisition or attire. He sought not power or possession or prestige or property or pay or pomp, but rather purity."

Before event-packed 1972, with its four awards, six overseas trips, scores of lectures, and Cassy's wedding, came to a close, Denis had one more major lecture to give, in Copenhagen, Denmark.

As his plane neared that city, the pilot found the weather too foggy to land and detoured to southern Sweden. After landing, Denis quickly boarded a ferry to Copenhagen, wondering if he would make the lecture on time. He was stunned to realize that he had neither the address of where he was to lecture nor the name of a contact person. Unfortunately, he'd been counting on someone meeting him at the airport. What was he to do?

Providentially, he met a pharmacist on the ferry who volunteered to phone his own hospital and inquire if there were posted notices announcing Burkitt's lecture. If so, they could find the location and time of the meeting. This was a fortuitous meeting with the pharmacist, for the idea worked well. Denis obtained the information he needed and arrived just in time for his lecture—to the surprise of all, for they had already announced that his plane had failed to land.

Momentous occasions? Yes, but greater ones were still to come!

*****

By 1973, data-gathering for his nutritional research had engaged Denis for six years. Although constantly reaping awards from previous contributions in the field of cancer, his focus of study and interest had now almost entirely switched from cancer to nutrition and Western diseases. Reflecting this change in medical emphasis, his voluminous medical writing up to 1973 included twenty-eight published articles on various phases of nutrition and its impact on disease. Of his twenty-two articles published in 1973 alone, a single lonely article on Burkitt's lymphoma testified to his former burning focus. His constant interest now was FIBER!

His determination to impart information in the affluent world meant an unbelievable schedule, answering requests to lecture, appear on television and radio, and be interviewed by magazines and newspapers. He saw but one way to popularize the benefits of fiber and healthful nutrition—to throw himself unremittingly into the controversial subject. And it was controversial! But disagreements, he felt, were not bad, for the media publicized these frays with increasingly meaningful exposure of the subject.

He began in January of 1973 by speaking at various British medical societies. On February 12, he presented his fiber-protective argument for bowel cancer at the WHO (World Health Organization) workshop of the International Agency for Research in Cancer. But he found he was fighting against odds. The fiber idea was still not at all popular in British medical circles.

His extensive traveling always meant a sacrifice for Olive. Fortunately this time, when he left on February 18 for a lecture tour beginning with Kabul, Afghanistan, and ending in Baghdad, Olive also made a trip. She went to stay with Judy and Philip, who were now teaching in Nairobi. His four weeks of subsequent travel meant getting up at three or four in the morning to catch planes. His schedule called for lectures and hospital visits in New Delhi, Calcutta, Poona, and Assam in India, Dacca in Bangladesh, and Katmandu in Nepal. The brief lecture-stop in Baghdad netted him a silver, embossed dagger inscribed with:

PRESENT OF IRAQI MEDICAL SOCIETY TO
MR. D. BURKITT
COMMEMORATING HIS VISIT TO BAGHDAD
18TH MARCH 1973

Back in England, he interspersed lectures and meetings with Hugh Trowell and other workers in this field. One unexpected honor was an invitation to speak at the British Nutrition Foundation (BNF) conference. Lecturing before this organization, which had initially turned down his article on fiber until Sir Ernst Chain interceded, he was exceedingly careful to give fiber facts and not antagonize his audience.

April 3 and Olive's birthday occasioned this diary notation: "Anxious thoughts may fill my heart but your presence is my joy and consolation." How pleased he was to be home with Olive for the celebration.

In May, the Royal College of Surgeons of Ireland made him an honorary fellow. While in Ireland, he spoke at his old medical school, Trinity College, Dublin and in his teaching hospital, the Adelaide. This excerpt about him written several years later, encapsulates Denis's reception at that time:

His oratory is direct, personal, almost unique. He lectures to popular audiences, to critical scientists, to irreverent medical students, to evangelical Christian groups, in great lecture theaters, in small rooms, on TV or video tapes, always with compelling and witty simplicity. Truly a genius, of a scarce pattern.

While in Ireland, during a lecture at the Galway Medical School, he asked if anyone would conduct a study on volunteers eating large amounts of potatoes. Being an Irishman and knowing that potatoes were an Irish staple in the past, Denis was curious to know the effect of these tubers on bowel transit-times. A young surgeon, John Flynn, undertook the study. Flynn, in turn, recruited twenty-five students and assigned them to eat two-and-a-half pounds of potatoes a day plus anything else they wished. This diet resulted in their passing large, soft stools with reduced transit-times. The students also lost weight, blasting the idea that potatoes were fattening. The fiber in potatoes was effective, indeed!

During his next trip to the United States, at the end of May, he lectured on fiber and colon cancer at Howard University, Massachusetts General Hospital, Columbia University, and at American pathology meetings in Detroit. From Chicago he flew in an executive Kellogg plane to Battle Creek, where company officials welcomed him and he spoke to their top representatives. This hectic three-week tour ended with appointments in Cincinnati, Pittsburgh and Morgantown.

At home again at The Knoll, Olive had a list of needed repairs about the house. The roof had been leaking, so Denis mounted a ladder and repaired it. The lawn certainly needed a good mowing—"excellent exercise"—which he enjoyed. A few ceramic tiles had come off the bathroom wall. As with his writing or lecturing, he worked on these menial tasks with energy and enthusiasm, for while doing them, he had the opportunity "just to think."

*****

Denis and Olive had been following the news from Uganda with some alarm since 1972, when the initial rejoicing at Idi Amin's rise to power began to wane. Amin had begun deporting the Indians, who, of course, were the business people and artisans, mechanics and carpenters. Often, the deportees' belongings were confiscated. Rumor was that, with the departure of so many key artisans and business people, everything needed repair, with resultant chaos.

Next, Amin asked many professors and British persons who held government positions to leave. What would become of their many friends still in Uganda? Michael Hutt continued to make his yearly visits to Uganda. He and Ian McAdam tried to salvage Makerere, but the outlook was grim. Ted Williams resolutely stayed by and carried on, undaunted, with his medical work.

During this time, Denis and Hugh submitted for publication their book, *Refined Carbohydrate Foods and Disease*, which had been years in preparation. Denis enjoyed his association with Hugh Trowell, for he was an excellent editor. It pleased Denis that Trowell was being invited ever more frequently to give nutritional advice and to lecture. Often they made appearances together. One additional honor came to Burkitt in 1973, the Gardner Foundation Award in Toronto.

✶✶✶✶✶

Not slowing down for a moment, Denis started 1974 with two overseas appointments, first to Ghana and Liberia, then to Miami for a conference of the American Nutrition Foundation. A quick trip to Belfast and Londonderry in March gave Denis and Olive the opportunity to visit Laragh once more with its new occupants, as well as to visit with old friends in Ireland.

One morning shortly after his return from speaking in Glasgow, Olive suggested that before he left for meetings in Portsmouth and Leeds, there were two things she wished he'd do.

Looking up from a sheaf of typewritten pages which he'd been proofreading, he said, "I'll do anything within reason. I can use a diversion."

"Wouldn't it be nice if you made a trolley to hold equipment for Judy's expected baby?" she asked. "You do such nice carpentry," she added, "and Judy would certainly appreciate it." Judy and Philip were now back from Africa, living in England again.

Denis smiled and said, "It's always your blarney that gets me to do what you want!" He put his stack of papers into a drawer. "Do-

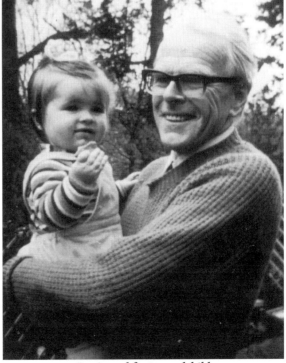

Denis and first grandchild.

ing a bit of woodwork will be a welcome relaxation after all this writing and lecturing. I need a change. Now, what was the other request?"

This one Olive really hated to ask. She looked at their old golden retriever sleeping in the hall, and said, "Don't you think it time to put Ranee down? It's been eight years since we brought her back with us from Kampala, and she wasn't a young dog then. It'll be the merciful thing to do," Olive finished, her voice trembling a bit. "The dog is really quite miserable."

Denis knew Olive was right, but this was a hard decision for him as well. "I can't do it myself. Ranee has been such a pet, like one of the family. I'll take her to a veterinarian."

Denis's respite at home was short-lived. Later in March, speaking at an all-day meeting on fiber sponsored by the Kellogg Company at the Royal Society of Medicine, he met considerable opposition from the millers. After his lecture, they attacked him. *How ironic*, he thought. *Here in England where most of the work on fiber and Western diseases has been done by various investigators, we seem to have the greatest opposition! I rarely have any criticism in the States. The U.S. media are always eager to disseminate our information.*

It was a relief to be well-received by the medical society in Washington D.C., where he spoke again on fiber and bowel cancer. From D.C., he flew to Lima, Peru for a whole week of lectures, followed by more in Brasilia and Rio de Janeiro. His talks on Western disease and fiber were well-received in each city. One more stop in Lisbon, and he was back home briefly, long enough to write a foreword for Cleave's updated book. He was about to publish *The Saccharine Disease*, at last. But this time Campbell's name had been left off as a co-author. Denis had persuaded Cleave to author the book alone.

Good news reached Denis in May. The Americans were considering fiber important enough to have an international conference in Boston devoted entirely to the subject. They asked him to participate with a presentation of his views.

June 10 was a joyful occasion with the birth of Judy's and Philip's daughter, the first Burkitt grandchild. Denis had managed somehow to finish the baby trolley in time, in spite of his impossibly-busy schedule. A second joyful occasion for Denis in June was an invitation from the British millers to deliver another lecture on fiber at their annual meeting. This time the millers were friendly and there was a reconciliation, concerning which Denis wrote in his diary: "I praise the Lord!"

The Kellogg Company sponsored a trip to Africa for Denis at the end of June 1974. He was able take Olive with him and to spend time again with Alec Walker in South Africa. He heard reports of Ted and Peter Williams at the Kuluva Hospital drawing blood specimens on 40,000 children for the massive Burkitt's lymphoma program. This project had taken them over two years and would not be completed for several years. The plan was to test for antibodies on the sera of those children developing the lymphoma in the next few years.

While still in Africa, they said a final, sad goodbye to the faithful Pastor Galiwango. It would be the last time they would see him, for his eventual fate under the Amin regime was never known.

Cassy and her doctor husband, Andrew, having decided on African mission service, left in August for what would become an eight-year total commitment to Kenya. Judy and Philip, in the meantime, having returned from Africa, settled in the small English village of Bisley. There Philip went into a successful nursery and landscaping business.

In the last three months of 1974, Denis made four overseas trips which included Mexico, the United States, Italy, India and Finland. On his far-flung travels, he always preached the fiber and Western diseases gospel. He was rapidly disseminating the word around the globe in both Western and Third World countries.

*****

Although Denis professed to understand little himself in the field of the microbiology of cancer, Burkitt's lymphoma was becoming a major cancer studied for chromosome changes. With constantly developing equipment and sophisticated techniques, scientists were now able to examine minute parts of the cell nucleus as it underwent division. They pondered the most basic portions which dictate all aspects of life—the chromosomes—during this stage of nuclear mitosis. Each of the forty-six, x-shaped human chromosomes had been identified, paired, numbered, and according to size, placed in groups.

Away back in 1960, an important discovery had been made in studying the malignant blood cells of chronic granulocytic leukemia. These leukemic cells had a minute, abnormal chromosome, subsequently called the "Philadelphia chromosome." From then on, scientists began searching cancer cells to find chromosomal abnormalities. In 1972, Manolov and Manolova reported the malignant B-lymphocytes of Burkitt's lymphoma had a longer chromosome 14 than normal. What was the significance?

Following up this lead, Zech, Haglund and co-workers, would report in 1976 a characteristic chromosomal abnormality in BL. They found the abnormally long chromosome 14 had resulted from the translocation of a small segment of the distal region of chromosome 8 to the distal end of chromosome 14. The same year, van den Berghe and his associates would find that the chromosome 8 segment in BL could also translocate to chromosomes 2 and 22.

Still later, in 1979, Croce, Shander and co-workers would find that the three chromosomes 2, 14 and 22, carried a focus for human immunoglobulins. Investigators identified translocations involving the same chromosomes 8, 2, 14, and 22, also in B-cell acute lymphocytic leukemia. With this information, Rowley speculated that the rearrangements resulted in proliferation and transformation of the lymphocytes in the cancers. What a complex picture was emerging! Little did Denis dream how far his one observation of an African child with an unusual jaw tumor would go in helping to open the whole field of cancer study.

*****

By 1974 and 1975, although Denis was no longer writing medical articles on various aspects of BL, there was one cancer in which he was especially interested, colon cancer, one of the Western diseases.

In 1975, Denis made six overseas trips. When in Edmonton, Canada, he filled one hiatus in his dietary research as he investigated the Eskimo diet. Olive accompanied him again to America when they visited the Blocksmas in Grand Rapids. His life was a whirl of activity.

A trip to Nairobi in June allowed him to spend time with Cassy and Andrew at their mission hospital in Kenya. Denis had expressed many years earlier that he hoped she might use her physiotherapy in Africa and someday go by car and plane with him on safari. He had his wish, as both Cassy and Andrew traveled with him on a road and air safari.

September 15, 1975 was a big day for both Denis and Hugh, as the first copy of their new book, *Refined Carbohydrate Food and Disease: Some Implications Of Dietary Fibre*, six years in the writing, arrived. Hugh had suggested the additional subtitle shortly before publication. It would show that their emphasis, as the main cause of these diseases, was fiber-depleted diets and not refined carbohydrates, specifically sugar.

This was the first book solely devoted to the dietary fiber theory and Hugh had extensively documented each of their arguments. Their friend, Sir Richard Doll, had written the preface, and as earlier promised, they dedicated the volume to Cleave. Hugh's chapter on diabetes was especially controversial to Cleave, for Hugh was first to submit fiber-depletion as one causative factor in the adult form of the disease.

As Denis pondered his successes and failures during the tremendously busy 1975, of one thing he was truly certain, his relationship with God. He wrote in his diary:

> Life is like a boat drifting down a river which flows at the end over a waterfall. The boat is our body. Flying overhead are helicopters offering a lifeline to any who will accept it. Many boats go over, but those persons holding to the lifeline are hoisted up to safety. Most

people are interested in the boat and not in the lifeline, the only thing that will matter in the end.

Even though Denis was striving to avoid unnecessary bodily suffering of millions, yet he always looked beyond the temporal to the eternal. "For what is a man profited, if he shall gain the whole world and lose his own soul?" *Does not medicine seek to save the body, at best lasting only a century, when eternal life is given little thought?* Denis pondered.

And what of his own future, now that he was fast approaching sixty-five? The Medical Research Council in London had turned down his grant request to continue his work. He was expected to retire.

Retire? Impossible! But what would his future hold?

17

"BURKITTISMS"

Since 1963, when Denis Burkitt gave his first international lecture at the M.D. Anderson Hospital in Houston, Texas, he had been on the lecture circuit, often giving thirty to fifty talks per year. Somewhere along the line, he began using original allegories to illustrate the points he was trying to underscore. These soon became an expected feature of his up-to-date scientific presentations. He found that many persons would approach him years after hearing one of his lectures to tell him that they still remembered his pictorial illustrations. Consequently, he came to believe that a picture was a far more valuable teaching tool than words, or even humorous illusions, though his lectures were also full of these.

Since Judy had an artistic bent for cartooning, he would often suggest the type of depiction he wanted and then use her caricatures in his lectures, with pointed, homespun comment. Since he'd spent so many years in Africa, it was only natural for him to think in terms of the African scene, and hence this early "Burkittism":

> If I should want to locate a dead elephant in Africa, I wouldn't part the tall grass to try to find it. I'd never find it that way. But there are always vultures flying around in the African sky, and they would be attracted to the elephant carcass (Fig. 1). So I should forget about trying to locate the dead elephant, and look for the obvious vultures, seen miles away, and follow them. Right beneath the vultures, I'd look around and soon discover my dead elephant.

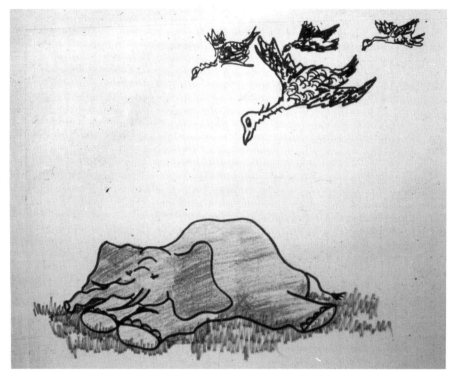

Figure 1

An investigator in medical epidemiology could use exactly the same idea. If two diseases are always closely associated (as vultures and dead elephants), it would be easier to locate the one that's more obvious and use it as a guide to the less obvious.

A medical example: most bowel cancers are believed to originate in benign polyps. There must be a common cause between the two. Polyps of the bowel (like the vultures) are infinitely more common than are malignant tumors of the bowel (the elephants). Yet, far more time, effort and money has been expended in searching for the cause of colon cancer than has been spent on finding the cause of bowel polyps. (Incidentally, the citizens of the countries that don't get bowel cancer, don't get bowel polyps either).

In other words, find diseases which are associated with the one you are interested in, and then choose the easiest one to follow up.

*****

Certain of Burkitt's mannerisms—occasional clearing the throat, blinking or coughing—never detracted from his message. He often accompanied frequent shifting of his weight from one leg to the other with a winning smile. Nor was it unusual for him to draw a humorous bit of information from history and imaginatively expand on it to make his point.

> In regard to hemorrhoids, or "piles," remember that during the battle of Waterloo, Napoleon had to go around on horseback inspecting his troops and army formations while suffering terribly from hemorrhoids. His mind must have often been more on his "piles" than on the strategy of the battle. If someone had put Napoleon on a high fiber diet, particularly bran, about six weeks before the Battle of Waterloo, he wouldn't have had to worry about his "piles."' He could have concentrated on the battle and might even have won it! We don't know if the outcome at Waterloo would have been different, but it's nice to question the possibility.

His Irish brogue, which he'd never tried to modify into proper Oxford English, captured his audiences, especially Americans, who enjoy an accent. Because Burkitt was a rapid talker one might miss an occasional word but never the gist of his message. One of his oft-used analogies was well-expressed by two of Judy's cartoons. (This is referred to in Chapter 16).

> Consider the picture of water running from a faucet, overflowing the basin beneath and flooding the floor (Fig. 2). Then we have two highly-trained, dedicated, highly-motivated gentlemen, with "A grades" all the way through college and medical school down on their hands and knees. Their sole purpose in life is keeping the floor dry, so they spend sixteen hours—eighteen hours—a day floor-mopping to get the floor dry. They have no time for their wives. They never see their families, because they've got to mop.
>
> Now, the water running from the faucet represents the cause of disease. The flood on the floor symbolizes the diseases filling our hospital beds, doctors' waiting rooms, and the operating rooms. Ninety-nine and two-thirds percent of money spent on medicine and health in North America goes for mopping floors—curative medicine. One-third of one percent goes toward turning off faucets—preventive medicine. Surely, we ought to be spending more time and money turning off the faucet!

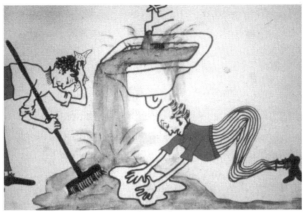

Figure 2

Any audience of physicians would have to agree that Denis was speaking the truth. However, many in the curative profession would begin to squirm as he continued his analogy.

> Now if I go into doctors' offices in North America, all four walls are plastered with framed testimonies of all floor-mopping courses they've attended, which makes them very good floor-moppers. Both before and after graduation from medical school, they spend much time learning and practicing effective methods of floor mopping, which cover all branches of curative medicine. They pay very little attention to turning off faucets. But unless they do

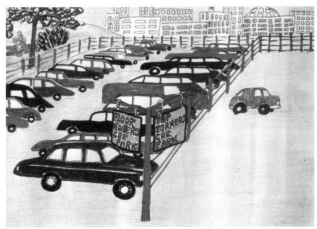

Figure 3

something to turn off the faucets with preventive medicine, it's a bit of a waste of time, spending all their time mopping the floor.

Then we have two car parks (Fig. 3). The car park for the floor-moppers are full of Lincoln Continentals, Cadillacs, and what-have-you. The car park for the tap-turners-off is almost empty. There's only one small car there, and it has a flat tire. This small car belongs to a nutritionist or health worker who is trying to prevent disease. [Denis and Olive have a Volkswagen]. We've got to have both the curative and preventive physicians, but there's no balance between the two groups of doctors at present.

*****

Burkitt always stood tall, with a military-like stance. When contemplating what to say next, his frequent mannerism was to put the tips of his spread fingers together and bring them up to his pursed lips. When beginning his favorite "taboo" topic, he'd look around and size up his audience. He, no doubt, was the world's best-informed lecturer on this "delicate" subject.

We know of no country in the world whose population gets hiatus hernia, diverticular disease, gallstones, bowel cancer, or coronary heart disease, if they pass large stools. All communities in the world who pass small stools, have high rates of all these diseases. That's only an observation, but it gives us reason to think. And of course we now know the major factor which is responsible for large stools is having adequate fiber in the diet. Today, there's endless research work available showing that fiber in the diet can be protective against diverticular disease, hiatus hernia and bowel cancer.

You see, researchers have gone into all sorts of chemistry, bio-chemistry, and molecular biology without ever weighing a stool. In fact, I had one experience in America which I'm unlikely to forget. I was speaking to the academics in the department of gastroenterology at a well-known university. I said to them, "You chaps know all about the gut. You make your living on the gut. You write papers on the gut. You write books on the gut. You hold conferences on the gut. You dream about the gut, and you're altogether experts on the gut." They sort of nodded assent.

I said, "I'd like to ask you one simple question before I lecture to you, if you don't mind. I just want to ask you, how much stool does the average American pass per day?"

And they looked at me in amazement, and they scratched their heads. I mean, they never thought of a question of that nature. The answers I received from a roomful of academic gastroen-terologists varied from six grams to two pounds. They'd never given the thing a thought. If I'd asked them some complicated question like the microscopic appearance of the duodenal mucosa of the colobus monkey, they could have written a whole essay on it. But to think of how much stool one passes—they'd never given thought to it. Isn't that amazing?

As has already been noted, one subject above all others that Burkitt preached was the *Priority Of Prevention Over Cure*. Not infrequently, he took hard but humorous cracks at the medical profession. As a surgeon and recognized scientist, he could get away with it!

If a shelf is fastened at an angle to the wall, any earthenware pots placed on it will inevitably tend to slide off and break when they hit the floor (Fig. 4). This predicament could be tackled in two different ways. Far the most popular and rewarding is to employ

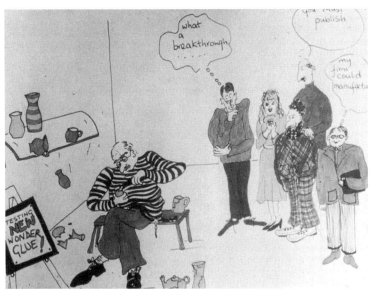

Figure 4

an acknowledged authority on repairing pots. In addition, this expert has invented a "new wonder glue." The broken pieces are mended in a manner not previously excelled. Every onlooker sees in this an opportunity for making a quick buck. Not surprisingly the chairman of the glue company is the happiest of all for he is excited at the prospects of increased profits.

But the question that should have been asked is "Why are the pots sliding off the shelf?" The obvious answer is that the shelf has been fixed at the wrong angle to the wall.

So a man comes along with the novel idea of straightening the shelf, dealing with the cause of the problem (Fig. 5). No longer do the pots slide off. The acknowledged expert pot-fixer is out of business. All the onlookers see their prospect of gain slipping away, while the chairman of the glue company is sinking into deep depression. But it is far better for the pots! Each of us, if we were the pots, would rather stay on the shelf than fall off and have the best surgeon in the area attempt to repair the damage.

*****

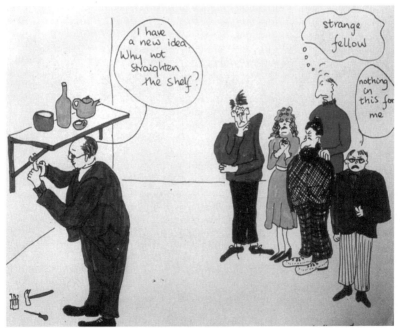

Figure 5

Burkitt, knowing human nature, and physicians in particular, enjoyed pointing out that sometimes there seemed to be a preference in the medical community for the complicated solution to a medical problem over the simple.

> If a puddle is forming where a kettle stands on a table, hypotheses must be made to explain the pool of water beneath it. The first observer pondering the situation suggests that the steam escaping around the kettle lid might create the pool of water (Fig. 6). A second more intricate, and consequently more acceptable theory, is that the steam from the kettle condenses on the ceiling and subsequently drips down onto the table, forming the puddle. A third idea is that the steam may condense on an overhead water pipe and then drip onto the table.
>
> No one suggests the simplest and consequently the least acceptable suggestion—there might be a leak in the kettle!

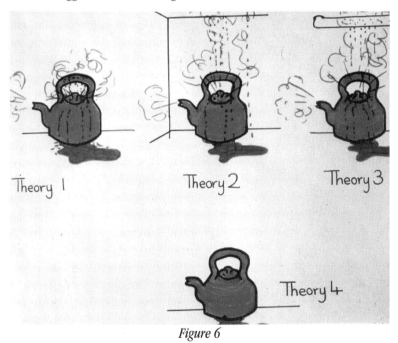

Figure 6

*****

Getting some "distance" from a problem in order to see it in its entirety (such as the causes of Western diseases) was something that Burkitt advocated.

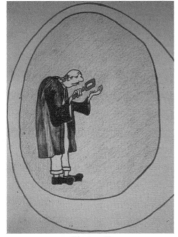

Figure 7

There are many ways in which a forest may be examined. Each leaf on the trees can be examined minutely through a microscope. Or the leaves of a branch can be examined in relation to one another. A still wider view can reveal how the branches are related to one another on the tree. But seldom is the relationship of the trees in a forest studied. Even less often is the forest viewed as a whole.

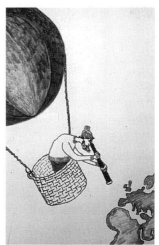

Figure 8

The different approaches are illustrated, first, by a learned professor viewing the particles of the cell through a magnifying glass (Fig. 7). He is contrasted with an investigator, like a man in a balloon viewing the trees and the forest, (Fig. 8), who stands back and views the problem as a whole.

*****

It is doubtful, when Denis asked Judy to draw the cartoon of a scientist in a hot-air balloon, that he ever thought of himself as being literally a passenger in one. However, this very experience was his and Olive's in Grande Prairie, Alberta, Canada (Figs. 9, 10).

Many years before, while lecturing at the Pritikin Longevity Research Institute in Santa Barbara, California, Burkitt had met a young cardiovascular epidemiologist, Dr. Hans Diehl. Diehl, a graduate of the Loma Linda University School of Health, had recently given repeated lecture invitations, accepted by Denis, to speak at the Coronary Health Improvement Projects [CHIP], which Diehl was conducting in various Canadian cities.

During his eightieth year, in 1991, Denis, with Olive, visited Grande Prairie for five days, giving ten lectures, two sermons at churches, holding press conferences, and also having fun. The city's host, Kenneth Fox, administrator of the Queen Elizabeth II Hospital, arranged a river jet boat trip on the Peace River, a helicopter

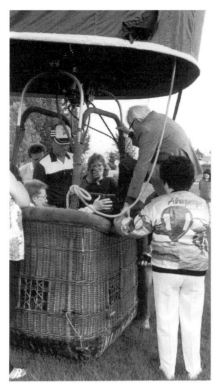

Figure 9

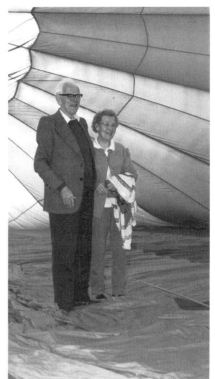

Figure 10

ride over the surrounding wilderness and Kakwa Falls, and also a hot-air balloon ride!

A Canadian tradition is to toast, with champagne, the passengers after their first hot-air balloon ride. They liberally toasted Denis and Olive with sparkling, white grape juice instead. The hospital medical staff, as well as the community, enjoyed their visit with Burkitt, whom they admired as a renowned physician and educator.

They marveled at his hardiness at age eighty and that their rigorous schedules didn't phase him. Their press release described him as the "conscience of the medical profession." They loved his typical, eyebrow-raising "Burkittism," such as, "Grande Prairie would be better off passing bigger stools than adding a new wing to the hospital." Denis also exclaimed in the interview:

> Health-wise, the only way forward is to go backwards. We all have stone-age bodies that haven't changed. But we are putting entirely different food into the tanks. If we are going to get rid of our major health problems in North America, we have to go back to the circumstances into which we were made to live. That means cutting down on our intake of fat, sugar and salt, and increasing

219

the amount of dietary fiber and complex carbohydrates we consume.

*****

On his frequent transatlantic flights (he estimated at least 100 of them during his long career), Burkitt usually traveled with little baggage. Often a single suit for the shorter trips sufficed. Variations came with different shirts and the addition or subtraction of a sweater-vest. In the winter, a padded field jacket often served instead of an overcoat. It is possible that he never owned a hat. Very much like his father before him, externals meant little. But the internal, the spiritual, always meant much. Occasionally, Denis found that he could weave a spiritual lesson into a medical research truth.

> *You See What You Look For!* If someone is not looking for a disease, he may never see it, although it's there all the time. This may be illustrated by one who is looking for the beautiful and sees the sunlight and lovely scenery. Another merely focuses his vision on the ground and complains (Fig. 11). The same scene is open to both, but the two see only what they are looking for.
>
> A second illustration of this point is that one can either focus the eyes on the "material things," represented by dust on the window glass (Fig. 12) and see nothing beyond, or he can look through the glass at a beautiful view and "spiritual realities."

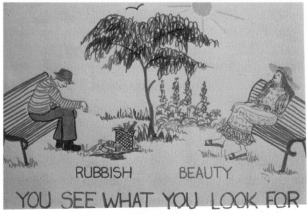

Figure 11

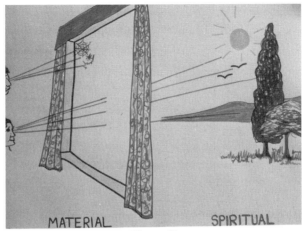

Figure 12

On another Canadian health crusade, directed by Dr. Diehl in Kelowna, British Columbia, a large crowd of CHIP alumni met Burkitt at the airport with a banner, singing a welcome song to the tune of "Clementine" (Fig. 13).

For once, Denis was speechless as he listened to the welcoming song, written by Rev. Albert Baldeo, an alumnus of CHIP. Burkitt, festooned with a lei made of fruits and vegetables, later preached on "Man—Carton or Content," at Rev. Baldeo's church:

> One of the fundamental errors in nutrition was the failure to recognize the role of fiber, which led to a deliberate policy of removing the outer, fiber-rich coats of cereal seeds. In the West, this was particularly evident in the endeavors to make whiter flour, while in the East the popular product was white rice. The "carton,"

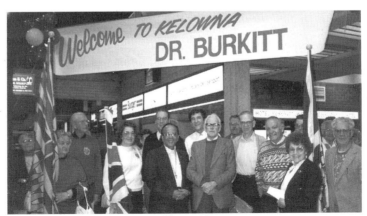

Figure 13

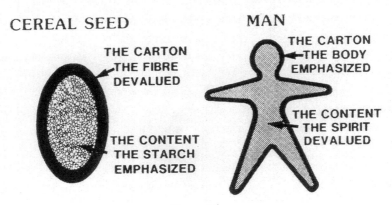

Figure 14

the coat with fiber, was discarded, and attention focused on the enclosed endosperm, the starch (Fig. 14).

Advances in scientific medicine and technology have led to another mistake in much of clinical medicine. So much can be effectively done for the ills of the body, or the "carton," that it now receives almost exclusive attention from physicians. The spirit, or the "content" is increasingly neglected or ignored....

When Diehl had asked Burkitt for his curriculum vitae (CV) for a medical society in British Columbia, he had written: "Tell them my CV is this: I'm a disciple of the Lord Jesus, and what a poor one at that!"

*****

One might wonder how Denis could retain his popularity while giving the medical profession a sound spanking. However, none could deny his unequivocal scientific truth, and by framing it in a humorous way, using imaginative parables, he blunted the blow. Precious few ever left one of his lectures angry or insulted. Rather, every honest person had to admire the man who could use such simple illustrations to present often overlooked, or unpopular basic facts. As Brian Kellock in *The Fiber Man* expressed it:

> Denis Burkitt's success as a communicator, whether lecturing on geographical pathology, his Christian faith, or fiber in the diet, stems from a total belief based on personal experience that what he is saying is true. But there is also that added quality which compels even those who disagree with him to pay attention, a

charismatic ability to communicate original ideas in a compelling, yet basic and often witty way.

At the close of a lecture, "War on Cancer with Analysis of a Failure," at the Health and Welfare Building in Ottawa, Ontario in 1990, this was his main thrust:

> If we are going to be dead honest, the treatment of cancer in the Western world has been a dismal failure. The problem is that most of our effort is directed toward early detection, treatment and molecular biology, none of which reduce the risk of cancer. According to Sir Richard Doll, there has been no significant improvement in survival rates from cancer since the early 1950's....

Then he launched into his statistical support of prevention of cancer through lifestyle changes, both dietary and exercise. The blame for escalation of Western diseases he placed on a failure to understand simple dietary factors.

> The millers took fiber out of wheat, because they didn't understand its valuable function. It's just like the surgical approach to many diseases has been, if something is not understood—take it out. I had my tonsils taken out at home, when a boy, by my uncle. In the past when we didn't understand tonsils and the immune system, we took them out. We didn't understand the appendix so we chopped it off. We went around nipping everything off because we didn't understand it. Often that has been the surgical approach....

Burkitt also hit strongly at basic research, having to find all the mechanisms and microbiology of cancer. It was interesting, he retorted, but it wouldn't *prevent* cancer. He compared the history of Admiral Gilbert Blane in 1775 ordering every ship in the British navy to carry lime juice to prevent scurvy. It was 150 years later that the *reason* lime juice prevented scurvy was discovered.

> If it had been today, researchers would have said, "Gilbert, my dear boy, you can't go giving lime juice to the navy. You haven't done a double blind study yet. You must hold off 'til we understand it."

Then he used one of his favorite allegories to illustrate the inequities between preventive and curative medicine.

Here we have a dangerous cliff with many people falling off, with broken legs and arms. There are two possible solutions to the predicament. We can either build a fence to prevent people falling off the cliff, or we can have a stream of ambulances at the foot of the cliff to pick up the injured. After being hauled off to the hospital by the ambulance and recovering, the fellow picked up, praises the ambulance driver (who, incidentally, gets three times the salary of a person building a fence). The fence-builder's work is more effective, but it's more popular in the medical profession to drive ambulances.

A favorite and effective way of ending a lecture, Denis used once more in this lengthy Ottawa lecture. Quoting the poet, Ogden Nash, he loudly finished, "We're making *g r e a t* progress, but we're headed in the wrong direction!"

In thanking Burkitt for his words of wisdom, epidemiologist Kenneth Johnson commented, "There is a quotation attributed to Bacon: 'Old wood is best to burn, old wine to drink, old friends to trust, old authors to read,' and I'd like to add my own: presenters who have been on the planet for a large number of years, to listen to."

Denis Burkitt's popularity and number of lecture requests were phenomenal, and these had continued unabated for over twenty-five years.

How many other physicians have held such a record?

18

HOW TO HANDLE HONORS

Retirement! Burkitt couldn't believe he was that old, for he certainly didn't feel like sitting back and folding his hands. Yet his appointment with the Medical Research Council was soon to expire with an enforced retirement at sixty-five. However, he had faith to believe that if the Lord wanted him to continue in his present work, He would provide as He had repeatedly in the past.

And Denis was not to be disappointed! In a talk with Wilfred Hamilton of the Kellogg Company in December 1975, Burkitt was assured of a supporting grant. This would cover not only an honorarium, but a secretary and an expense account for photographic slides used in lectures. Hamilton, in the name of Kellogg's, promised all of this with the understanding that Burkitt would in no way promote their cereal products.

When Michael Hutt, Professor of Geographical Pathology at St. Thomas's Hospital Medical School in London since his return to England in 1970, heard of Burkitt's imminent retirement, he immediately invited him to join his department. He provided a small room for him off his own office, and gave him an appointment as an honorary senior research fellow at St. Thomas's. The Lord *did* provide.

Burkitt, on one of his most recent African trips, had seen his old friend Ted Williams finishing an important research project with Dr. Guy de-The', from Lyon, France. For several reasons, the National Cancer Institute and the International Agency for Research in Cancer had selected Ted as part of the team to work on an important lymphoma project. Not only was his district around the Kuluva Hospital

225

in the West Nile District of Uganda an area of high density for the cancer, but Ted had kept meticulous records in his own cancer registry for years.

Williams had also worked with Dr. Pike a few years back on the "clustering" phenomenon of the disease. Moreover, Ted and his brother, Peter, were fluent in several local languages. The African people considered them as "two of us." This newest, ambitious BL project would be a monumental epidemiological study, which would really require the ingenuity of these medical brothers to ensure success.

The Henles in Philadelphia had discovered that the Epstein-Barr virus, originally recovered from Burkitt lymphoma tissue, also caused infectious mononucleosis and was a ubiquitous virus worldwide. However, they realized that evidence was still lacking to pinpoint the EB virus as the actual cause of the tumor. Its presence in the tumor could be incidental, although almost invariably the EB virus was found in each cultured biopsy of the cancer from these African children.

The Henles, therefore, envisioned a massive collection and storage of frozen blood serum samples from every child in a heavily endemic area. As the subsequent months and years passed following their initial serum collection, whenever a participating child developed the tumor, a second serum sample was to be taken. Then the paired blood specimens were to be examined for a rise of EB virus antibody in the second serum sample.

Researchers had found EBV antibodies in nearly 100% of African children, the infection possibly transmitted from infected mothers. The mothers' habit of pre-chewing all food given their babies was thought to be the mode of early transmission of disease to babies. Because every African child had EBV antibodies, the Henles realized it would be necessary to show that children developing BL had reacted *differently* from other children to a second infection with the virus. That difference might be *age at the time of infection,* the *degree of infection*, or the *response to the virus.*

What work this study entailed! When the team arrived at a locality, they held a public meeting in which Ted or Peter explained the purpose of the testing. They measured into a large plastic container, red-colored water equivalent to the total blood volume of a child. Then they filled a two-milliliter syringe from the colored water, demonstrating the relatively tiny amount of blood which would be drawn from the children. This convinced parents that the procedure was not dangerous.

Subsequently, the Williams brothers had registered about ninety-five percent of all children, two to eight years-of-age, in the area. They had drawn their blood and made blood smears for malaria detection. The tubes of blood had been placed immediately in insulated coolers and, within a few hours, refrigerated. The following day the team had collected the sera from the blood clots and stored these in a freezer. The labeled tubes of serum were finally shipped in liquid nitrogen for storage in

Lyon, France. From February 1972 to September 1974, they had drawn a total of 42,000 serum samples!

Later, Denis heard the results. Between 1973 and 1977, fourteen cases of BL developed among the children who had previously been bled. Ten of these fourteen BL children had unusually high EBV antibody titers when compared with the antibody levels in the sera of matched, normal African "control" children. Furthermore, these ten children also had unusually high antibody titers on their original sera samples, suggesting that children with heavy primary exposure to EBV were at increased risk of developing BL. This intensive study strongly supported a causal relationship between the Epstein-Barr virus and Burkitt's lymphoma.

However, it was experiments undertaken by Drs. Thomas Shope and George Miller of the Yale School of Medicine that gave final proof that the EB virus did, indeed, cause the lymphoma. Shope and Miller injected the virus into marmoset New World monkeys. While some of the animals merely produced antibodies to the virus without becoming ill, others rapidly developed fatal lymphomas. This clearly showed that the EB virus was the causative agent.

While Drs. de-The', Ted and Peter Williams were conducting their massive study, the political situation in Uganda was becoming increasingly tense. By 1975, the Idi Amin government had threatened to deport all Britons. Uganda had for many years been a largely Christian country. Now, not only the educated, but Christians as well, had been targeted by Amin, a poorly-educated Moslem. With deportation since 1972 of Indian artisans, along with the business-engaged foreigners, the country was deteriorating badly. Ted Williams at Kuluva was constantly being threatened.

One day, while he was hearing reports of Amin atrocities and of the thrilling rescue of foreigners held hostage in the Entebbe airport, two burly black policemen appeared at his hospital. Ted feared for his cancer records and quickly decided his strategy.

"I'm sick and tired of always being threatened!" he exploded, shouting, "furthermore, I'll quit! I'll go on strike until you stop harassing me!" Stunned, the policemen hardly knew what to do. They retreated. Ted ranted on saying, "I'm tired of all the road blocks and being threatened with machine guns." He continued his tirade until the two men left.

It wasn't long before Ted received an urgent call. A voice asked, "Why are you on strike?"

"I've had enough and am tired of being constantly threatened," Ted answered.

"Oh, please don't leave," the voice on the phone pleaded. "We need you here. You're helping us so much." He had put his point across. It was the last time he had trouble personally, but Uganda, as a whole, continued to disintegrate.

By mid-1975, the Makerere Medical School was limping along, having lost much of its well-trained faculty. In spite of several visits by Michael Hutt and Ian McAdam to encourage the faculty, the future was unpromising. For years the school had been accredited with the General Medical Council of England, which periodically sent examiners from Britain. But this year Amin had refused to allow entrance of the examiners into the country, so the medical school lost its accreditation. Only medical degrees conferred prior to 1975 would henceforth be recognized in the United Kingdom.

*****

If Denis was amazed by the end of 1972 to have received eleven awards or honorary degrees, he had experienced nothing yet. As a humble man, his attitude remained unchanged. He reflected on his honors in this way:

> I look back with deep gratitude to God over a life filled with many joys and the privilege of seeing some apparent fruit from enterprises in which I have been involved. I am profoundly thankful for the numerous tokens of recognition of supposed achievement that have been bestowed upon me in the form of awards and honorary degrees. It would be hypocritical to pretend that these had not brought pleasure, but I can say with the utmost sincerity that I would have gladly declined some if instead they could have been given to those who have worked closely with me and to whom I owe much.

One of his greatest thrills came in 1974 when he was awarded the CMG, Companion of the Order of St. Michael and St. George. It was bestowed by Queen Elizabeth II herself. The award was given principally for distinguished overseas service. In priority it ranks lower than a knighthood but senior to most other decorations.

What an exciting time for the Burkitts! Rachel, living in London at the time, volunteered to drive Denis and Olive to Buckingham Palace in her Mini Austin. Of course she also wanted to attend the affair. As they drove into the palace grounds, big, black limousines nearly engulfed the little Austin. Denis, in his tails, and Olive in a long gown, got out of the car while Rachel found a parking place. As the three were ushered into the palace, they heard muted band music coming from a great hall.

While Olive and Rachel sat as spectators, Burkitt and others receiving awards were given instruction. They must know the proper procedure when the queen arrived and how to bow upon acceptance of the decoration. For the investiture, they cued up in order. A person standing next to the Queen read a list of the accomplishments of each participant. To receive from the Queen's hand the decoration was a thrill Denis would never forget as he stepped backward, scroll in hand, and made the second designated bow.

*****

Because Burkitt had made it his practice not to turn down an opportunity to speak if he could work it into his busy schedule, he usually made at least four transatlantic flights a year. On one occasion, in St. Louis, he lectured on the geographical distribution of cancers to a conference of medical students from twenty different American medical schools. His interesting way of lecturing, mixed with a good dose of Irish humor, appealed to the young people. On an impulse, they asked him to give their banquet speech that evening as well.

Filling an extemporaneous speaking request had never been difficult for Denis. As he looked at their earnest young faces with a lifetime of medical practice ahead of them, he decided to risk talking in a spiritual vein. He stressed that their contributions to medicine would depend more on their attitude than on their ability, to their motives rather than their methods, and on character rather than cleverness. He recited John Oxenham's famous poem:

> One ship sails east and another west,
> While the self same breezes blow.
> It's the set of the sail
> And not the gale
> That bids them where to go.
> Like the waves of the sea,
> Are the storms of the fates,
> As we journey along through life.
> It's the set of the soul
> That decides the goal,
> And not the storms and the strife.

In his conclusion, he stated that "man is more than a biological creature; he was made in God's image," He almost held his breath. How would these young people in a materialistic world respond? They rose together, giving him a standing ovation for his forthrightness. Afterward, many students crowded around him, asking, "Why don't any of our professors talk to us like this?"

*****

Was it possible? Their last daughter, Rachel, was to be married on July 10, 1976 to Dr. David Maurice. Physicians had run in the Maurice family for six generations, but what was even more unusual was that their family practice had always been in Marlborough. So unusual was this Marlborough medical practice of six generations that the *Guinness Book of Records* cataloged it. Once more the Burkitt family readied The Knoll for the event as Denis and Olive prepared for the large number of guests attending. Of course Rachel would not be going to Africa as Judy and Cassy had, for it would never do to break the Maurice tradition of medical practice in Marlborough!

*****

Ever since the San Diego American Cancer Society conference and his lecture on fiber and colon cancer (published in *Cancer*, 1971), Denis had felt somewhat guilty. He knew that his friend Alec Walker in South Africa had done the original work on the subject, but Walker had failed to publish a paper on it. Consequently, Denis's presentation, although quoting Walker, had been viewed as the first on the causal relationship between colon cancer and fiber, but it had never been Burkitt's intention to usurp Walker's rights.

Eight years later, in 1978, as a delegate to the International Conference on Colorectal Cancer held in New York, he had his opportunity to publicly disclaim originality. There he gave full credit to Walker for the fiber-colon-cancer concept. In his lectures, he had always been careful to honor both Cleave and Trowell for their

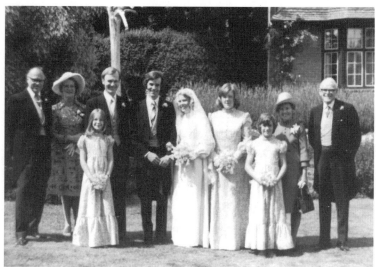

Rachel and David Maurice's wedding with corresponding immediate families.

original contributions. In fact, he still felt very much like a spokesman for them in proclaiming their views, as well as his own.

Later in 1978, when Denis came home from work one day, Olive was waiting for him. "Someone rang for you. He had a very cultured voice, but he wouldn't leave a message. I told him when you'd be in."

Before long, the telephone rang again, and Denis answered it to hear a "cultured man's voice" saying, "This is Peter Ashmore (not using his full title, 'Rear Admiral Sir Peter Ashmore'). The Queen would like to know if you will be free on February fifteen to have lunch with her."

"Surely you must have the wrong telephone number." stammered Denis, unable to think of anything else to say.

"You're Mr. Burkitt?" the voice persisted. "The queen *does* want you to lunch with her on the fifteenth of February."

Denis, flustered, was thinking, *No matter what I've planned, I can't refuse an invitation from the queen! This is not really an invitation, but a royal command.* "Yes, of course, I'd be delighted to come," he said. Hanging up the phone, he quickly drew his appointment book from his inside coat pocket and flipped the pages. "How could I be so fortunate! The date is open," he sighed with relief.

While Olive waited for him to identify the mysterious caller, she had been joined by Judy and Rachel.

"I've been invited to lunch with the Queen," he said. "Now don't smile. It's true!"

The girls, by then quite accustomed to the many prestigious people their father knew, were not completely surprised. They began chanting the nursery rhyme, "Pussy cat, pussy cat, where have you been?"

Denis laughed heartily and answered, "I've been to London, to see the Queen!"

In a few days, the official embossed invitation arrived. There was no doubt, he would "see the Queen." He told no one at the office about the appointment. When the day arrived, he put on his overcoat and went out the door. He had previously decided that if anyone asked where he was going, his answer was ready, "I'm going to lunch with the Queen." Naturally, it would be taken as a joke. It was a little disappointing when no one asked!

Since he was working at St. Thomas's, about a mile from the palace, he simply walked. Of course, he arrived far too early, being "terrified" of coming late. So he paced up and down past the sentries outside Buckingham palace for a while. Finally he showed his ticket to the guard at the gate, who said, "Walk on."

Passing through the big gate, he felt quite conspicuous as the sole pedestrian on the walkway to the palace. He was ushered into a room to hang up his overcoat and was then met by Sir Peter Ashmore, who introduced him to several other distinguished guests from various occupations. They included a newspaper editor, a professor of music, an author, an actor, and a high government official. It was hardly a private luncheon.

After the guests visited among themselves and selected from a variety of drinks, Peter Ashmore ushered them into the formal dining room. The Queen and the Duke soon entered, and the luncheon began. Afterward, the royal pair chatted privately with each guest before retiring to their quarters. As Denis returned to his office, he hoped he could remember how to describe everything to his curious, waiting womenfolk at home. For a loyal British subject, this luncheon was a truly memorable highlight!

*****

As the years rolled by, Denis garnered many additional honors. In 1973 he received the Gardner Foundation Award in Canada and a fellowship in the Royal College of Surgeons in Ireland. He also received a fellowship in the Royal College of Physicians in Ireland in 1976. The British Medical Association tendered him their gold medal in 1978, and the Bristol University granted him an honorary M.D. in 1979.

On one of his trips to America in 1978, he attended an M.A.P. Missionary Conference, and after he'd gone to bed in his hotel, Ray Knighton phoned him. He told Denis that the Board of Governors was inaugurating the Ralph Blocksma Award, to be given annually to someone making an outstanding contribution to medical missionary work. They had chosen Denis as the recipient of the first award.

"Ray, you can't mean it!" he remonstrated. "I've never served as a medical missionary except for acting as Chairman of the Board of Governors at the Mengo Hospital. There are so many really worthy missionary doctors."

"You've been chosen, Denis," Knighton repeated, "and it's impossible to get the board together again. If you refuse the award, it won't be given at all, and that would be a great disservice to Ralph," he argued.

Since there was no one Denis would rather see honored than Ralph, he submitted to the decision. Ralph and Ruth were attending the M.A.P. Conference, knowing nothing about the award to be given in Ralph's honor. That evening, the master of ceremonies first called Blocksma to the platform and announced the inauguration of the award, which was applauded. Then to Ralph's surprise and delight, they called Burkitt to come forward as the first recipient. Ralph hugged his dear friend while the audience stood, applauding. A wooden plaque with a large brass plate bore the image of Ralph, and below, the words:

PRESENTED TO DENIS PARSONS BURKITT, BY M.A.P.
INTERNATIONAL, IN RECOGNITION OF DEDICATED AND

COMPASSIONATE SERVICE TO THE PEOPLE OF THE
WORLD THROUGH CHRISTIAN MEDICINE, JUNE 4TH, 1978.

There was more to come a few days later. Denis spoke at the Annual House of Delegates Meeting of the Christian Medical Society. After the dinner, Sid Macauly, a regional representative rose to speak. Turning to Burkitt, he said, "Denis, we have chosen you to receive the 'Servant of the Year' Award."

Denis was not only surprised, but full of consternation as he looked out on the audience of dedicated missionaries. He knew in his heart that any one of them was more deserving of the honor. He feared the only reason for the award was that his name was known scientifically. There was nothing he could do, however, but accept as a token of their love the sculpted porcelain bowl with draped white towel on a wooden base. A brass plate bore the inscription,

SERVANT OF THE YEAR, 1978

*****

Even though there was no ceremony connected with his being made an honorary fellow in 1979 of his old University, Trinity College, yet it was a thrill and a satisfaction. This honor caused him to search his memorabilia file, which included some of his father's correspondence, until he found what he was looking for, a letter with the heading, *Trinity College, Dublin.* It was dated November 7, 1929, fifty years earlier. It had been written to his father by Denis's adviser during his first year at the university, when Denis was struggling in the engineering course.

Dear Burkitt:

The enclosed gives all information. [Grades enclosed].

Don't blame me if he gets stuck and loses his 10 guinea fee, or if he fails his exams in 1930 and loses the year.

I suppose you have thought of it. But I daresay he will pull it off. All the same it is a risk.

I hold this up till I have seen his marks. The April fee (10 guineas) must be paid shortly before he sits for the term finals. The October fee will fall due shortly after.

Yours sincerely,

Luce

Denis smiled. *That was a while ago, and now they want to elect me as an honorary fellow. If I had just had some inkling of the future, it might have saved me some worry and perspiration at the time!*

There was no scroll. No presentation ceremony. The secretary just informed him of the citation bestowed. But to be an honorary fellow of Trinity College was more prestigious than receiving an honorary degree. He learned that only one other living medical doctor had been so distinguished. Theoretically, there were some advantages also. He could get a free meal in the dining hall at any time, and in addition, a bed and breakfast in the guest quarters for nothing.

Also in 1979, Denis was more than pleased to attend and witness Captain Cleave receive two much-deserved gold medals at the Royal Naval Hospital in Gosport, South England, where he had once worked. Vice Admiral Sir John Rawlins, Medical Director of the Royal Navy and member of the council of the Royal Institute of Health, presented him the Harben Gold Medal. At last, his years of dedication to the improvement of health in the recognition of Western diseases was being recognized. This was indeed an honor, as previous recipients had been men like Pasteur, Lister, Gowland, Hopkins, Fleming and Flory.

On the same occasion, Sir Douglas Black, President of the Royal College of Physicians, and Mr. Selwyn-Taylor, Senior Vice President of the Royal College of Surgeons, bestowed on Cleave the Gilbert Blane Gold Medal for outstanding service to naval medicine. Denis knew how very much this day meant to Cleave, who had struggled for years under a cloud stalwartly clinging to his ideas in the face of great opposition. Denis wrote an article describing the occasion, titling it, "Ridicule Replaced by Recognition."

Later in the year, Denis learned that Ted Williams was at long last leaving Uganda and settling not too far from him in England. The previous few years Ted had worked under great pressure, never knowing what the next day might bring. A fractured hip led him to leave Uganda at last. It was probably the hardest decision of his life, for he had hung on in spite of adversity, since this was his dedication and the life he really loved. For years, he had kept remarkable records of all cancer cases, his outstanding interest and contribution being the Burkitt lymphoma cases. Now, this chapter of his life was closing. However, with his move to England, he was not too far from Denis, and the two old friends enjoyed occasional visits.

*****

In spite of the recognition he'd already received, Denis's big year was 1982, when he was granted three awards and honors. By now, far more acknowledgment of his contributions to science had come than he had imagined possible. He learned that in the United States, a board of scientists had just elected "Professor M. Anthony Epstein and Dr. Denis Burkitt to jointly receive the Bristol-Myers award for distinguished achievement in the field of cancer research." They would be the first foreign recipients of this prize. About the same time he learned that the University of Leeds would confer on him an honorary Doctor of Science degree.

When traveling in the United States a couple of months later, Denis was told at his hotel that a caller from New York had repeatedly tried to reach him but would not leave a message. His curiosity was shortly satisfied. He received the phone message that he had been selected for the distinguished Charles Mott award donated by General Motors Corporation for his studies in cancer causation and prevention. By now he felt totally astonished and undeserving of all the impending honors.

Denis appreciated the thoughtfulness of the Bristol-Myers presenters, who invited Olive to join him for their special occasions. The pharmaceutical company started their presentation and press coverage in England, since both Epstein and Burkitt were from the United Kingdom. The press conference began with an elaborate luncheon served in the elegant Chandos House, an extension of the Royal Society of Medicine in London. *The luxurious reception in beautiful surroundings*, Burkitt thought, *were of marked contrast to the primitive circumstances of his work in Africa which had ultimately lead to the occasion.*

On the other hand, he reflected, *This is a fitting recognition for the magnificent work done by Tony Epstein and his colleagues. His studies on the EB virus have been the most fruitful project in the whole field of viral oncology today.* Then rather apologetically, he decided to himself, *I presumably have been included for having been, in a sense unwittingly, the initiator of this development. Whereas I left the field of cancer study a decade ago, Tony has been contributing constantly during this whole time.*

For his acceptance speech on the Bristol-Myers occasion in London, he made a characteristic Burkitt analogy.

> When a space rocket is launched, you have to have a launching pad from which the rocket is launched. The pad isn't a great scientific accomplishment, but it has to be there to get the highly sophisticated triumph of modern engineering off the ground. My work proved to be the launching pad for the Epstein-Barr virus rocket. It took far more skill and knowledge to make the rocket than the pad, but the rocket needs the pad, and I accept the position of being the launching pad.

Having enjoyed a harmonious, personal friendship for years, Denis and Tony emphasized the different nature of their contributions in the cancer field when they met with the British press.

True to his nature, after he and Olive were offered first-class plane fares to New York for the American portion of the Bristol-Myers celebration, Denis immediately requested that they travel by economy class instead. He asked if the money saved by the difference in price of the tickets could be donated to a retired missionary doctor who had been helpful in his work. This, however, he was informed, was not feasible in view of tax writeoffs. So, for the first time, the Burkitts basked in what he described as the "ridiculous luxury" of first-class air travel.

Taking out a notepad and pen as the plane taxied for takeoff, he busied himself for a few minutes. "I have just calculated the cost of our combined first-class round-trip flights per minute," he announced to Olive. "It's costing the exorbitant figure of £2 (about $5.00) per minute!"

"It's frightfully expensive to go first-class," she agreed.

As they gained altitude, even before the seat-belt signs had been turned off, he did a bit more figuring. "Our sponsors have paid more for our trip during just the last twenty minutes than the cost of my total research grants for the first eighteen months of the lymphoma project," he said, incredulously. Denis had always been proud of how far he could make money stretch.

Olive, he soon noticed, was loving the exquisite meal service, including the white linen place mats under the china dishes, in contrast to the usual plastic dinner-tray service of the economy class. *I'm afraid, because of my frugal nature,* Denis admitted to himself, *I've too often denied her even reasonable comfort, let alone luxury.*

On their arrival at the Kennedy Airport, a chauffeur with a black Lincoln Continental limousine whisked them off to the Waldorf Astoria. When they were settled in their room, Olive remarked, with some hesitation, "I wouldn't mind having a drink of orange or lemon juice."

"If this were an ordinary hotel," Denis said, "I'd simply drop a coin in a machine and get a cold canned drink. But this is the Waldorf Astoria." He rang for room service and ordered a couple of glasses of orange juice. When a waiter promptly delivered the juice on a linen-draped tray, Burkitt couldn't resist asking, "I say, what is the price of the juice?" Although he didn't have to pay the bill, he couldn't believe it. Five dollars! *Such a waste!* he thought.

Over their glasses of orange juice, he and Olive reminisced, comparing their present luxurious accommodations to that of many previous third-rate hotels where they'd stayed through the years. And they had to agree that their happiest memories were of times spent in comparatively simple circumstances. At the same time, they wondered at how Providence had led them to this moment and humbly thanked God for His goodness.

The next day, Burkitt was occupied with newspaper, radio and television interviews. The following morning, the day of the actual presentation, Denis happened to read from his Bible the account of Christ's transfiguration before His disciples. As a bright cloud enveloped them, the disciples heard only God's voice saying, "This is My beloved Son, in whom I am well pleased. Hear Him!"

Contemplating the scene, Denis made a warning note to himself in his diary: "The clamor claims and consciousness of material pressures and pursuits stifle the voice of God." He had always been attentive to God's leading in his life, and he determined anew to be an obedient servant of the Lord.

About 400 cancer-research scientists with their wives or husbands attended the presentation luncheon. Burkitt recognized and spoke with many old friends, including several who had been at the Kampala lymphoma conference in 1966, just before they moved their home from Africa.

He could hardly believe how his first research endeavor from such small beginnings had blossomed. The silver medallion presented to him was inscribed with:

BRISTOL-MYERS AWARD,
DISTINGUISHED ACHIEVEMENT
IN CANCER RESEARCH.

He was also handed a generous check. In his New York acceptance speech, he again used a typical Burkitt analogy.

> My contribution to this cancer research might be likened to a boy gathering sticks to light a fire to boil water in a kettle. Should others come along, pour on oil and fan the flame causing a prairie fire, the blame would be laid on the shoulders of those who fanned the flame, not on the boy who lit the fire. My little fire has been blown up into a spreading blaze by Tony Epstein and others. As the flame-fanners in the analogy deserve the blame, so the fanners of my flame deserve the credit.

Their return flight to England was again luxurious. Even Denis thought how nice it was to have a limousine meet them at the London airport. And when the chauffeur delivered them to their very door past midnight, he had to admit that they might otherwise have had difficulty in finding transportation home at that late hour!

✳✳✳✳✳

Six weeks later, accompanied by Olive, Judy and Philip, Denis drove to the University of Leeds for an impressive ceremony conferring honorary degrees on six august personages. The University Chancellor conferring the degrees for the occasion was Her Royal Highness, the Duchess of Kent. Prior to the presentation ceremony, the honored recipients and their wives were invited to tea with the Duchess. In speaking with Denis and Olive, the Duchess recalled that she and her husband had met them twenty years earlier when Uganda was receiving its independence.

Following the tea, the six honorees donned their respective robes and academic hats and were escorted to their places in the colorful procession. With the Chief Marshal leading. members of the staff, professors, deans, representatives of religious bodies, local authorities, the presenting professors, the Vice-Chancellor, and finally the Chancellor, the Duchess herself, marched in.

An appropriate University professor presented with a short speech each distinguished person to receive his honorary degree, declaring the person's accomplishments. Burkitt's presenter was Professor Gerald Richards, an old friend and a fellow member of the Christian Medical Fellowship. Professor Richards led him to the platform as the Duchess conferred the Doctor of Science degree. Following the ceremony, the Duchess invited the awardees, their relatives and special friends to a formal dinner over which she presided. In her speech, she mentioned each of the honorees by name with appropriate accompanying comments. The festivities of the entire afternoon were conducted with utmost dignity and warmth.

✻✻✻✻✻

Olive took Denis's dinner jacket from the closet. "You've not worn this for years," she commented. "The Charles Mott Award function in America certainly has to be a very formal occasion, since it specifies that a 'dinner jacket' be worn!"

"Usually these award affairs in the States haven't been that formal," Denis said. "I wore an ordinary suit for the Bristol-Myers occasion." Eyeing the dinner coat, he asked, "Do you recall when I bought that jacket in Uganda?"

"Yes, I remember our finding an advertisement in the paper for a dinner outfit with coat and trousers. It was just when you needed one for a function in South Africa," Olive recalled.

"A real bargain, too," Denis added. "Only three or four pounds. And I can still use it. Certainly no need to buy a new one when I wear the suit so seldom. The small darned place on the left shoulder will never be noticed."

The morning before their leaving once again for America, Denis read aloud to Olive the words from Deuteronomy 8:13, 14 and 17:

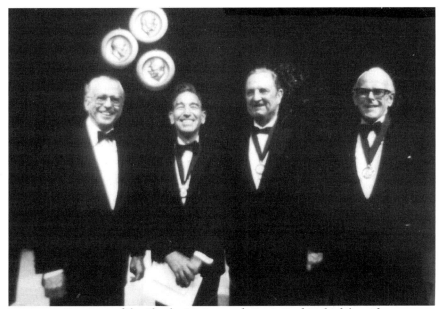

Honorees of the Charles Mott award: Denis Burkitt (right), with Drs. Stanley Cohen and Howard Skipper. Left, General Motors Chairman.

> When your herds and flocks increase, and your silver and gold and all your possessions increase too, do not become proud and forget the Lord your God who brought you out of Egypt.... Nor must you say to yourselves, "My own strength and energy have gained me this wealth," but remember the Lord your God: it is He that gives you strength to become prosperous....

"I couldn't be reading anything more fitting this morning," he exclaimed. "I've certainly never cared for money, but regardless of what comes to us, we must remember it is God who has given us everything."

On their arrival once more at New York's Kennedy Airport, they couldn't miss a large placard inscribed with *"Burkitt."* Upon identifying themselves, a chauffeur led them to a Cadillac limousine, for this time it was the General Motors Corporation which had sponsored their trip and was conferring the award. They were driven to the St. Regis Hotel for accommodation in New York during a series of press and television interviews.

The following day they were taken to Washington D.C., where the presentation was to be made. While the press again interviewed Denis, Olive was given a tour of the White House. After luncheon at the University Club, the other two recipients, Dr. Howard Skipper and Dr. Stanley Cohen, with Denis, were driven to the National

Institutes of Health in Bethesda. Here, each gave a thirty-minute summary of his scientific contribution.

Finally, the presentation itself took place in the evening at the State Department auditorium, where three gold medals were displayed in their black velvet-lined boxes on the platform. The Union Jack with the Stars and Stripes on either side, represented the respective countries of the honorees.

Following a preliminary speech by the Chairman of General Motors, the three recipients were again introduced by scientists familiar with their work. Standing beside Denis was a senior official from the British Embassy. The two Americans had their respective Congressmen standing with them. The General Motors Chairman placed a heavy gold medal suspended on a wide blue ribbon around each honoree's neck.

In the long reception line, Burkitt felt he hadn't shaken so many hands since their daughters' marriages. At the formal dinner, he and Olive sat with the President of General Motors and his wife; Colonel Frank Borman, former astronaut and his wife; and Mrs. Kettering, daughter-in-law of the self-starter inventor. She had visited in the Burkitt home in Uganda twenty years earlier, when his cancer studies were just beginning to attract world attention. Mr. Braithwaite, the British diplomat who had stood with him during the presentation, completed the table.

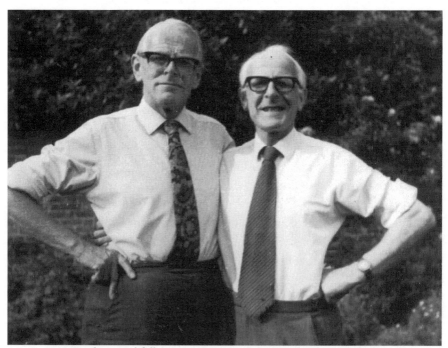

Brothers and fellow surgeons: Drs. Denis and Robert Burkitt.

As Burkitt ate the sumptuous dinner that evening, he thought again of how Providence had led him from insignificant beginnings in North Ireland to this present unexpected zenith.

Later in this eventful year, however, something befell the Burkitt family that made them all stagger a moment in contemplating God's plan and direction.

19

THE POTTER AT WORK

It was a time of togetherness and joy for the Burkitt family as they gathered around the dinner table at Judy's and Philip's house. Rachel and her doctor-husband David were not there, because she had just given birth to their first child, a son. After five years of marriage, this was an event to be especially celebrated.

"Now David has a son to carry the family tradition one more generation," Philip said, referring to the Maurice family's medical practice of six generations in Marlborough, recorded in the *Guinness Book of Records*. "When this son becomes a doctor, he'll be the seventh generation practitioner of the family in Marlborough, an unbeatable record!"

Judy excused herself to answer the telephone as they passed dishes of steaming food and began serving themselves. She returned in a few minutes, and from the expression on her face, they knew something dreadful had happened. "It was Rachel," she said, haltingly. "The baby—Edward—is a Down's baby."

There was sudden, painful silence. Denis looked at Olive, tears brimming her eyes. He had a heavy aching in his throat. *I would gladly have some fatal illness myself if I could spare Rachel and David this sorrow,* he thought.

Finally Judy broke the agonizing silence. "We can't question God or doubt His wisdom. We must thank Him for considering them worthy of bearing this burden. It will be up to us all to treasure little Edward and support Rachel and David with our love and encouragement." Everyone knew she was right. They must make adjustments, and all had hearts of love for the new little baby, who would be every bit as precious as Judy and Cassy's children.

As the news spread about little Edward, letters and many long-distance telephone calls enveloped them with expressions of sympathy, love and understanding. From the first inkling of the problem, both Rachel and David accepted their baby with adoring love. The prayer group to which they belonged immediately assured them that they would gladly share their joys, anxieties and responsibilities.

Denis could not but observe, *just as fortune and success tend to engender jealousy, so suffering and weakness tend to bring out all that is good. Has not the shameful, humiliating and agonizing death of the Son of God on a criminal's gibbet brought untold blessing to unnumbered multitudes throughout the ages down to our family today? Did not the Apostle Paul write that God has chosen the weak things of the world to confound the mighty? That's how it will be with our Edward.*

They had planned to give Edward the middle name of "Burkitt" to carry on the family name. But since he would likely never have a family himself, they decided to give him the second name of "Samuel," meaning "gift of God." He would become a special object of love for the whole family.

Denis and Olive especially appreciated Morris West's best seller, *The Clowns of God*, as he put these words into the mouth of Jesus when referring to a Down's child. (The "she" in the text has been replaced with "he").

> I know what you are thinking. You need a sign. What better one could I give than to make this little one whole and new? I could do it; but I will not.... I gave this mite a gift I denied to all of you—eternal innocence. To you he looks imperfect, but to me he is flawless.... he will never offend me, as all of you have done. He will never pervert or destroy the work of my Father's hands. He is necessary to you. He will evoke the kindness that will keep you human.

*****

Denis maintained a good relationship with the millers during the years when the question of fiber was resting with the COMA committee. They had even invited him and Olive to a reception at the prestigious Mansion House. As Denis was busily talking to various millers there, Sir Joseph Rank, the President of Rank-Hovis-McDougal, England's largest milling corporation, visited with Olive.

"At home, we accept and follow the advice of your husband," he said, "but we don't yet accept it in the industry." Perhaps he'd been reading Denis's and Hugh's second book on nutrition, *Western Diseases: Their Emergence and Prevention*. It had been released in March 1981 and had caused considerable stir in the media with extensive coverage.

This second Burkitt-Trowell book had thirty-seven contributors from all five continents, testifying to the rising interest in nutrition worldwide. Southerby, the great international auctioneers, shortly chose it to be included in a time capsule, selecting it among other books which they considered of key importance for this century. When the capsule would be opened fifty years hence, it would then be determined if the various books' predictions or trends had indeed been valid. Of course, the capsule's content by then would have become quite valuable and worthy of auctioning at a good price.

Finally, also in 1981, the British COMA committee was ready, after *eight long years*, to make a report on the status of fiber. Nearly a decade earlier, the milling industry had flatly refuted Burkitt's report relating fiber-deficient diets to Western diseases.

Very little was really accomplished in improving Britain's nutrition for many years. Not until 1979 had the Royal College of Physicians set up its own committee to consider the medical aspects of dietary fiber. But in the fall of 1980 it published a report emphasizing the importance of fiber in the diet.

So it was, a year later, that the COMA report also stressed the importance of fiber in bread and strongly recommended that the millers make whole-wheat bread more available to the public. About two months later a meeting convened at the Royal Society in London to consider these recommendations. This was a meeting Denis and Hugh did not want to miss! Two anonymous white-haired gentlemen found seats in the audience, hearing the warmly-applauded recommendations of the committee, including these items:

- Nutritional education should stress the value of bread as a good source of dietary fiber and nutrients.

- An increase in dietary fiber would be beneficial.

- Whole-wheat bread should be available in restaurants.

- Labeling of bread should include information as to dietary fiber content.

None in the audience felt more gratified than the two old friends, who sat in obscurity that day. They realized that their time committed to activating this general dietary change in the whole country had not been in vain. Nor was the trend for increasing fiber in the diet limited to the United Kingdom. FIBER had long since become a "password" in many other Western countries. The British media popularized the committee recommendations immediately.

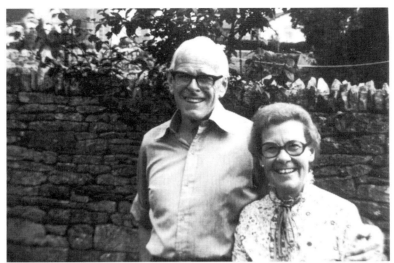

Denis and Olive celebrate their fortieth wedding anniversary (July 28, 1983).

Before long, copies of a best-selling diet book recommending fiber-rich foods for weight reduction, flooded the market, with over a million copies sold in a couple of months. Unfortunately, Burkitt regretted, *the author gave no credit to the instigator of the concept, Hugh Trowell, who had published this idea in medical literature two decades earlier.*

He thought back to his own 128-page paperback book, *Don't Forget Fiber In Your Diet*, published in 1979 for the lay public, with Martin Dunitz. It had been profusely illustrated with diagrams and colored pictures. He recalled how it had attracted magazine, newspaper, radio and TV interviews in Britain. The interviewers often asked what he thought of "Dr. ——'s diet." He was always careful to emphasize he was not promoting that doctor's diet or a "Dr. Burkitt's diet!" The American version of the book had a title which Dunitz thought more suitable for Americans, but which Denis disliked: *How To Eat Right To Keep Fit And Enjoy Life More*. Within three years, the little book had appeared in eight languages, attesting the growing interest in health and dietary fiber around the world.

Once the British millers became really interested in fiber, they began experimenting in the production of a marvelous new food called QUORN. They invited Denis to test this new product before introducing it on the market. Rank-Hovis-McDougal had developed it. By using fungi, they had been able to turn carbohydrates into protein. The conversion rate of 1:1, far surpassed the 20:1 rate at which animals convert vegetation into meat.

From the viewpoint of conserving energy, this new food proved to be tops. By adding various flavorings—chicken, ham, beef—it provided an acceptable meat substitute. Its meaty texture and a protein content the same as beef, but free from cholesterol and fat made the new product popular with many.

*****

In 1977 Denis was delighted when Hugh Trowell was invited by Senator McGovern's Senate Select Committee on Nutrition and Human Needs in the United States to serve as the lead-off witness for its hearings. Hugh had earlier been invited to dietary conferences on fiber in Edinburgh (1972) and Stockholm (1974, 1976). But his wife Peggy's growing incapacity made it possible for him to accept very few overseas invitations for many years.

Few people knew of Trowell's influence on the diets used by Nathan Pritikin at his Longevity Center in Santa Barbara, California. Pritikin, not being a physician, had come under considerable attack for his recommendations of diet and exercise for certain chronically ill patients. Trowell and Burkitt inspected Pritikin's institute. They were able to endorse his Spartan diet and methods, for he and his physician-staff were getting amazing results in patients with diabetes, hypertension, coronary heart disease, and obesity. Pritikin had initially blamed excessive fat in the diet for Western diseases, but Trowell persuaded him of the protective role of dietary fiber as well. Both Trowell and Burkitt participated in conferences at Pritikin's Center in 1975 and 1976.

Senator George McGovern had been a guest speaker at the second Pritikin conference which Trowell had co-chaired. Consequently, in 1977, McGovern invited Trowell as a dietary expert to the Senate Committee which recommended the first radical changes in the American diet. When this committee investigated the role of dietary fiber in Western diseases, they asked Trowell to introduce the subject, seeing that fiber research had originated in Britain. At the committee hearings, he compared American and African diet and disease patterns. He cited the Pritikin diet at the Longevity Research Institute, for which he had provided consultation. The McGovern committee at last proposed dietary goals for the American public, goals which Trowell endorsed.

Hugh Trowell was continually making additional contributions to nutrition research. Because the *Cumulated Indices Medicus*, did not at first reference "fiber," a literature research on the subject was very difficult. So Trowell developed his own laborious bibliography of 1,038 references, *Dietary Fiber In Human Nutrition (Bibliography)*. He published it with the help of the Kellogg Company in 1979, and it became most helpful to future investigators of the subject.

In 1985, yet another volume, *Dietary Fibre, Fibre-Depleted Food and Disease*, came from the editorial pen of Trowell with co-authors Burkitt and Kenneth Heaton. As with previous books, this one also had multiple contributors—thirty-two in all. Its authors discussed at length the developing newest concepts of dietary fiber.

Then, in 1988, Denis accompanied Hugh Trowell to the United States, where they were honored guests at the George Vahouny International Conference of Dietary Fiber in Washington D.C. (The passing of Hugh's invalid wife enabled him to travel once more). There Burkitt and Trowell met Alec Walker of South Africa. At a conference banquet attended by nutritionists from around the world, Trowell was presented with a beautiful citation. It read:

> In recognition of the efforts of Hugh Trowell in bringing the importance and benefits of dietary fiber to the attention of medical practitioners, research scientists and the general public, we officially recognize the contribution of Hugh Trowell to science, medicine and the arts of healing.

Walker and Burkitt were presented similar citations. This was a high point in the lives of all three men.

The following year, 1989, the British McCarrison Society, a professional association promoting sound nutrition, determined to honor Trowell at a special dinner in honor of his 85th birthday. For the occasion they asked Denis to write a booklet on Hugh Trowell's life and contributions to medicine and nutrition.

During its preparation, Denis sent the manuscript to Hugh, for he wanted the information to be accurate. The manuscript came back heavily marked by Hugh's trusty editorial pen. Denis made the corrections suggested by Hugh and resubmitted it to him for final approval. However, Hugh returned it again, heavily edited. The same thing happened once more. This was not like his old friend, and Denis became concerned that at the dinner celebration, Hugh might even stand up and make further corrections during its presentation.

However, only a week before the birthday when he was to be honored, Hugh suddenly died. In his last letter to Denis, he'd written, "As one grows older, one has to learn to accept that God progressively removes the faculties, one by one." Denis replied with the encouraging thought that, as the Apostle Paul expressed it, while the outward man is progressively perishing, the inward man can be renewed day by day.

In reviewing and writing about his dear friend's life, Burkitt had realized anew the depth of Hugh's dedication. As a medical student at St. Thomas's on a full scholarship, Hugh's chief had warned him not to go to Africa, as it was unlikely he could do any good medical work there. Sixty years later, his old medical school inaugurated the Hugh Trowell Lecture, proof that his many years in Africa had not been fruitless.

*****

Yet another honor for Denis. In 1984, Princess Ann conferred on him an Honorary Doctorate of Science from the University of London. Olive, with Cassy and Andrew on home leave from Africa, were able to attend the function.

Daughter Rachel, over the years learned so much in caring for her handicapped son, Edward, that she developed a ministry to other people. She now had two additional children, a boy and a girl. Feeling she might share some of her experiences as a help to other parents of children with Down's syndrome, she

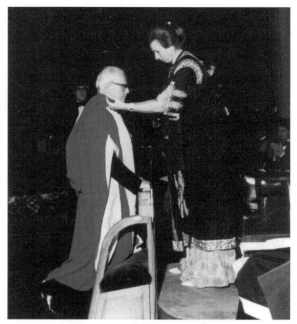

Princess Ann bestows CMG honor.

wrote an account of caring for her loving little son. It was published in the April 1987 issue of the *Journal Of The Christian Medical And Dental Society*, circulating in seventy-eight countries.

A doctor in Australia, upon finding his first grandson a Down's child, became utterly despondent. On his return from the hospital where the baby was born, he chanced to pick up the journal containing Rachel's article, "A Response to Handicap." It so encouraged him that he wrote a poem titled "Edward" which appeared in the next issue of the journal. Rachel was pleased that little Edward's life was being used by God.

*****

The year 1989 was especially busy for Denis. Six invitations came from Ireland to speak to local gatherings of doctors in unpretentious hotels around the country, invitations he greatly enjoyed filling. The South American branch of the Kellogg Company invited him and Olive to South America. He, with three other scientists from America, were to talk on fiber, diet and health. Their trip included Caracas, Venezuela, and Rio de Janeiro and Sao Paulo, Brazil. as well as Mexico.

They were both invited in 1989 to Paris, where Denis was to be inducted into the Academy of Sciences, a scientific body that had been created in 1666. Until recent years, most of its honorees had been French, but more recently the Academy included British, Russian, American, Italian, Japanese and German scientists.

The ceremony was one of the most colorful they had witnessed. It was held at the Institute de France, a famous rotunda designed by Cardinal Mazarin in 1663 and completed in 1684. A council member of the Academy, Professor Jean Barnard , who had once visited Kampala, had nominated Burkitt to this elite body. For the occasion, Academy council members wore black suits trimmed on the lapels and trousers with gold braid.

Those about to be admitted to the Academy, including Burkitt, lined up in the entrance to the rotunda. Olive and other guests were ushered to seats in a semicircle inside the auditorium where they were introduced to the Prime Minister, Paul Rocard. The name of each scientist was called out as he went forward on the platform. A resume of the honoree's work was read in French with an instantaneous translation into earphones used by foreigners in the audience. After the reading of individual accomplishments, the President of the Academy handed each a medal and a citation.

At the conclusion of this part of the ceremony, all marched down steps lined by uniformed soldiers beating drums and sounding bugles. But this was not the end of the festivities. Buses next provided transportation to the Palaíse de l' Élysée, the President's residence where the honorees were ushered into a reception room hung with lovely tapestries. The thirty men being inducted into the Academy formed a semicircle in front of President Mitterand, who gave a short speech and then shook hands with each. After the tapestries were drawn, all sat down to a buffet luncheon. Since neither Denis nor Olive understood French, trying to make conversation with participants and guests proved a bit awkward at an otherwise exciting occasion.

A particularly joyful event that same year, one where they surely felt more comfortable, was a special dinner at which Burkitt was honored by the town council of Enniskillen. The town fathers presented him a plaque and gave Denis and Olive a beautiful and memorable voyage on Lough Erne. He found it especially nice to be recognized in the town of his birth.

Denis took advantage of the occasion to invite two friends from their Africa days to share a grand tour of Ireland, something he himself had never before indulged in. A disappointment on the tour was Mullaghmore, the favorite vacationing spot of his childhood. Mullaghmore was now full of tour buses, and of people drinking beer, eating ice cream and littering everywhere. He determined, regretfully, never to return.

One remaining event highlighted 1989. Having once received the Charles Mott Award from General Motors, Denis got an invitation each succeeding year to attend the function and applaud the new honorees. He and Olive had never returned for such a program, but when the 1989 invitation arrived, Denis got an idea. He would like to take Cassy to the affair. She and Andrew had just returned permanently to England for the further education of their children after eight years' service as missionaries in Africa. She had never been to America. So Denis sat down and wrote a letter to the General Motors committee saying that his wife couldn't attend with him and asking if he might bring his daughter instead. After some hesitation, the committee agreed.

Denis and Cassy stayed in the Mayflower Hotel in Washington, D.C. She, in her lovely long dress, was able to accompany her father in his stipulated dinner jacket to the glittering affair and get a firsthand taste of how Denis himself had earlier been honored.

True to his ingrained thrifty pattern, Denis had exchanged the first class air tickets from General Motors for economy class on the transatlantic flight. This saving enabled him to procure round-trip air tickets as far as Denver. He felt it would be a shame if Cassy, on her first American trip, could not see something of the States. They flew to Denver, where a member of the Christian Medical Society entertained them in his home. From there they boarded a train to San Francisco so she could thoroughly enjoy the scenery en route. In San Francisco, she was able to visit friends from Africa who lived in the vicinity.

*****

Although Denis "retired" a second time in 1988, he didn't slow down but continued to make at least four transatlantic trips a year. Having their three daughters and families fairly close, he and Olive considered a real blessing. When

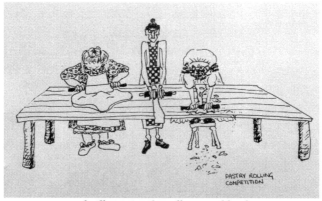

Judy illustrates the village cookbook.

Hartwell Cottage had been vacated in Judy's village of 800 people, she had urged that her parents buy this historic stone house in Bisley, just opposite her house.

After Judy and Philip returned from their two-year stint in Africa, in spite of his teaching credentials he really wanted to make landscape gardening his career. So, with Judy's encouragement, Philip took a one year course and afterward set up his own business in Bisley. He shortly became the village's biggest employer of laborers, sometimes as many as thirty. For five years, Philip earned a silver award at the prestigious Chelsea Flower show.

After their three children went to boarding school, Judy worked as a teacher in the local school. She also enjoyed youth work at the church, brought meals to the elderly, and took an active part in village events. For a church-related fund-raiser, she exercised her artistic bent, illustrating a neighborhood cookbook, for which she also collected recipes.

Cassy's husband, Andrew, a family physician, for several years after their return from Africa acted as a prime mover in starting a hospice for the terminally ill in their area. They erected a building, and because he was skilled in plumbing and electrical wiring, used these talents for this hospice project. Cassy daily utilized her physiotherapy training in their town, which was about eight miles distant from the Burkitt's village.

For Denis's eightieth birthday, February 28, 1991, Cassy wrote a poem, which her three children along with Judy's three and Rachel's two, took turns reciting at the family celebration.

ODE TO PA

1911 was uneventful,
Or so historians say,
But Denis was born in Ireland,
By Lough Erne, he learned to play.

He had devoted parents
And a sister too,
But younger brother Robin
Was the best friend that he knew.

Their upbringing was loving
And reas'nably straight-laced!
Cycling, fishing, not parties—
And paper, not girls, he chased!

251

At Trinity in Dublin city
Medicine he eventually read,
His faith and facts they blossomed
On bacon and eggs he fed!

Then on, to become a surgeon
And meet Olive, his lovely wife,
The World War came and went
Painful partings a fact of life.

He felt led to work in Africa,
So in 1946,
Leaving expectant wife in Ireland,
He went out into the sticks.

It was with the Colonial Service
That Denis to Uganda was sent.
At first to work up-country,
Later to Kampala he went.

But since Olive and baby daughter—
Judy was her name—
Joined that up-country station
Life was never quite the same.

His work as a general surgeon,
Church commitments and lecturing too,
Meant life was fulfilling and busy
With colleagues—a very good crew.

Not being girl-crazy when younger
This time must surely be!
Olive had two more daughters
Surrounded by women was he!

'Twas in Denis Burkitt's nature
To inquire about what he saw.
He developed an important interest
In a child's cancer of the jaw.

This led to exciting study—
Long safari, as well.
To the lymphoma being named "Burkitt's"
Most heads, not his, would swell!

With international recognition
And a place in history
He and Olive returned to England
To work for the MRC.

His questions "why" and "wherefore,"
His approach to global disease,
His contacts, research and colleagues,
Epidemiology did please.

Returning fiber to your food
Bran flakes, in bread and stew,
He studied stools of every race
And loved looking down the loo!

The medical world loved "Fiber Man"
His lectures had them in stitches,
He received awards around the globe,
But was never interested in riches.

He continued his simple lifestyle
His bath of one inch, no more!
Porridge for his breakfast
And fat is shown the door!

And so "prevention is better"
And "cheaper by far than cure,"
Was the gospel he preached worldwide
To nations both rich and poor.

Sons-in-law, three, nearby,
And nine grandchildren to boot
He still makes the odd "bookcase,"
Watches "fillums," and now computes!

This man has many qualities
Too many to name by far—
Love, faith and generosity,
All part of our much loved PA.

*****

In August, 1992, Denis and Olive enjoyed a memorable experience at Trinity College's 400th anniversary celebration, to which they were especially invited. For the occasion, the Burkitts were accommodated in a beautifully furnished apartment converted from the *very rooms* in which he and his Number Forty Christian Union friends had met for prayer sixty years earlier. Denis Parsons Burkitt had come full circle. His name, on this occasion, was listed with other renowned Trinity graduates: Jonathan Swift, George Berkeley, Edmund Burke, Samuel Beckett, Rowan Hamilton, Robert Graves, William Stokes, and *Denis Burkitt*. But Denis, writing in his diary that morning, had a different preference. He quoted Luke 10:20 "Rejoice, because your names are written in heaven."

*****

Two additional honors were yet to come to Burkitt. In 1992 he was inducted into the Royal College of Surgeons of Canada. However, in January, 1993, the capstone award was given him in Philadelphia's Franklin Institute. Here he received the American equivalent of the Nobel prize, the Bower Award gold medal and a monetary gift of $373,000. Its citation read:

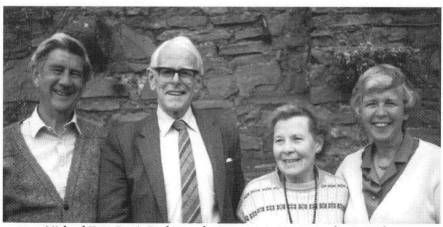

Michael Hutt, Denis Burkitt and wives visit in Hutt's Garden in Wales.

For innovative and creative research, under extremely difficult circumstances in a tropical developing region, leading to the establishment of a virus-cancer linkage in the widespread childhood disease that has become known as Burkitt's lymphoma and leading to the redirection of cancer research and treatment throughout the world. For his inventive and methodical documentation of factors that explain the geographic distribution of disease among world populations. For his advocacy of the hypothesis implicating a deficiency of dietary fiber as a fundamental cause of health afflictions in the industrialized world and for his humanitarian devotion to the health of mankind.

The foregoing citation really well-summarized Burkitt's medical contributions, but if anyone asked him regarding his accomplishments, he always downgraded them all with a statement such as:

In both the lymphoma and fiber research, what I did, without meaning to, was initiate all kinds of work by other people. I didn't do much, but my findings sparked much research by others. That all proved to be worthwhile. My work was a catalyst more than anything else. The number of papers that have been written on the lymphoma [around the world] has been incredible.

Tony Epstein and I both attended the conference in Naples in 1983 to celebrate the twenty-fifth anniversary of the discovery of Burkitt's lymphoma. By that time, molecular biologists swamped the conference. All that kind of stuff meant nothing to me at all. In 1989, there was a conference in Oxford to celebrate the twenty-fifth anniversary of the Epstein-Barr virus. They asked me to speak, but really I could understand nothing of what was going on in the conference. It was all over my head.

These honest remarks came from a man who had diligently turned out over 300 scientific papers and seven books!

The fact is that the unique tumor, Burkitt's lymphoma, has *sparked or contributed* to investigation in five areas of medicine: geographical pathology, virology in human cancer, chemotherapy of lymphomas and leukemias, immunology of cancer, and molecular biology, specifically, chromosomal translocations in human cancer.

255

As for his *popularizing* fiber deficiency and a refined, rich diet as the cause of Western diseases, his work has been monumental in turning the eyes of the world to focus on this problem.

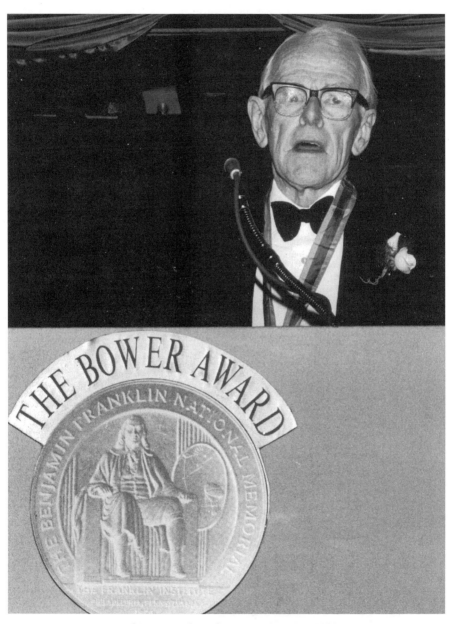

Burkitt responds to the Bower Citation, 1993

Only a "catalyst?" But what if there had been no "catalyst?" Thousands of research projects have blossomed in cancer and nutritional research as a result of his keen observation, persistence, energy, industry, and farsighted intuitiveness. The productive research of others has ultimately rested on the foundations laid by this humble, God-fearing, and yes, frugal, Irishman. This is true, even though he often said of himself, "The Potter worked on poor clay indeed!"

EPILOG

His research work, his medical and spiritual writings,
his informational and humorous lectures, his God-filled
sermons, his incessant travel, his worldwide friendships,
are over.

**Denis Parsons Burkitt passed to
his rest in England on March 23, 1993.**

*****

SELECTED BIBLIOGRAPHY

Bray, Elizabeth. *Hugh Trowell: A Biography*. Unpublished manuscript.

Burkitt, D.P. 1951. *Primary Hydrocele and its Treatment. Review of 200 Cases*. Lancet (England) 1: 1341–1347.

Burkitt, D.P. and Burkitt, R. 1952. *Acute Abdomens-British and Baganda Compared*. East Africa Medical Journal 29: 189–194.

Burkitt, D.P. 1958. *A Sarcoma Involving the Jaws in African Children*. British Journal of Surgery 46: 218–223.

Burkitt, Denis, and O'Conor, G.T. 1961. *Malignant Lymphoma in African Children: A Clinical Syndrome*. Cancer (USA) 14: 258–283, March–April.

Burkitt, D.P., Oettgen, H.F., and Burchenal, J.H. 1963. *Malignant Lymphoma Involving the Jaw in African Children. Treatment with Methotrexate*. Cancer (USA) 16: 616–623.

Burkitt, D.P., Williams, E.H., and Eshleman, L. 1969. *The Contribution of the Voluntary Agency Hospital to Cancer Epidemiology*. The British Journal of Cancer 23: 269–274.

Burkitt, D.P. 1969. *Related Diseases—Related Cause*. Lancet (England) 2: 1229–1231.

Burkitt, D.P. and Wright, D.H. (editors). 1970. *Burkitt's Lymphoma*. Edinburgh: E. and S. ivingstone.

Burkitt, D.P. 1971. *The Aetiologogy of Appendicitis*. British Journal of Surgery 58: 695–699.

261

Burkitt, D.P. 1971. *Epidemiology of Cancer of the Colon and Rectum*. Cancer (USA) 28: 3–13.

Burkitt, D.P. and Trowell, H.C. (editors). 1975. *Refined Carbohydrate Foods and Disease*. New York: Academic Press.

Burkitt, D.P. 1982. *Where Are You Going?* Richardson, Tx.: Christian Medical Society.

Burkitt, Denis P. 1989. *Trowell*. London: The McCarrison Society.

Burkitt, Denis P. *Man, Carton or Content?* Richardson, Tx.: Christian Medical Society.

Cook, Paula J., and Burkitt, D.P. 1971. *Cancer in Africa*. British Medical Bulletin. 27:14–20.

Croce, C.M. 1986, Dec. *Chromosome Translocations and Human Cancer*. Cancer Research (USA), 46: 6019–6023.

Dalla-Favera, R., Martinotti, St., and Gallo, R.C. 1983, 25 Feb. *Translocation and Rearrangements of the c-myc Oncogene Locus in Human Undifferentiated B-Cell Lymphomas*. Science (Wash. D.C.), 219: 963–967.

de- The, G., Tukei, P.M., Williams, E.H., Bornkamm, G.W., Feorino, P., and Henle, W. 1978, 12 Aug. *Epidemiological Evidence for Causal Relationship between Epstein-Barr Virus and Burkitt's Lymphoma from Ugandan Prospective Study*. Nature (England) Vol. 274, No. 5673: 756–761.

de- The, G. 1984. *Epstein-Barr Virus and Burkitt's Lymphoma Worldwide: The Causal Relationship Revisited*. Burkitt Lymphoma Symposium.

Epstein, M.A. 1956. *The Identification of the Rous Virus: A Morphological and Biological Study*. British Journal of Cancer 10: 33–48.

Epstein, M.A. 1964, 1 Feb. *Cultivation in Vitro of Human Lymphoblasts from Burkitt's Malignant Lymphoma*. The Lancet (England): 252–253.

Epstein, M.A., Woodall, J.P., and Thomson, A.D. 1964, 8 Aug. *Lymphoblastic Lymphoma in Bone-Marrow of African Green Monkeys (Cercopithecus Aethiops) Inoculated with Biopsy Material from a Child with Burkitt's Lymphoma*. The Lancet (England): 288–291.

Epstein, M.A., Henle, G., Achong, B.G., and Barr, Y.M. 1965/ *Morphological and Biological studies on a Virus in Cultured Lymphoblasts from Burkitt's Lymphoma*. Journal of Experimental Medicine, 121:761–770.

Epstein, M.A. 1985. *Historical Background; Burkitt's Lymphoma and Epstein-Barr Virus*. Burkitt's Lymphoma: A Human Cancer Model, 17–27.

Fenoglio, Cecilia M., and Lefkowitch, Jay H. 1983, Sept. *Viruses and Cancer*. Medical Clinics of North America, Vol. 67 No. 5: 1105–1125.

SELECTED BIBLIOGRAPHY

Geser, A., de- The, G., Lenoir, G., Day, N.E., Williams, E.H. 1982. *Final Case Reporting from the Ugandan Prospective Study of the Relationship between EBV and Burkitt's Lymphoma*. International Journal of Cancer 29: 397–400.

Glemser, Bernard. 1970. *Mr. Burkitt and Africa*. New York: World Publishing Co.

Gregory, J.R. no date. *Under the Sun*. Nairobi: The English Press.

Henle, W., Henle, G. and Lennette, E.T. 1979. *The Epstein-Barr Virus*. Scientific American, 241: 48–59.

Henle, Werner, and Henle, Gertrude. 1981, Nov. *The Epstein-Barr Virus-specific Serology in Immunologically Compromised Individuals*. Cancer Research 41: 4222–4225.

Hutt, M.S.R. and Burkitt, D.P. 1986. *The Geography of Non-infectious Disease*, Oxford: Oxford University Press.

Hutt, M.S.R. 1970. 6 Mar. *Cancer in Uganda—1900–1970*, The Fifth Albert Cook Memorial Lecture (UMA), given at Makerere Medical School.

Kellock, Brian. 1985. *The Fiber Man*, Tring, G.B.: Lion Publishing Corp.

Klein, E., Ernberg, I., Masucci, M.G., Szigeti, R., Wu, Y.T., Masucci, G., and Svedmyr, E. 1981, Nov. *T-Cell Response to B-Cells and Epstein-Barr Virus Antigens in Infectious Mononucleosis*. Cancer Research 41: 4210–4215.

Morrow, R.H., Gutensohn, N., and Smith, P.G. 1976, Feb. *Epstein-Barr Virus-Malaria Interaction Models for Burkitt's Lymphoma: Implications for Preventive Trials*. Cancer Research, 36: 667–669.

O'Brien, Brian, 1962. *That Great Physician: Sir Albert Cook of Uganda*. London: Hodder & Stoughton.

Pattengale, Smith and Gerber. 1973, 14 July. *Selective Transformation of B Lymphocytes by E.B. Virus*. The Lancet (England): 93,94.

Pike, M.C., Williams, E.H., and Wright, B. 1967. *Burkitt's Tumour in the West Nile District of Uganda 1961–5*. British Medical Journal, 2, 395–399.

Purtilo, David T., and Klein, George. 1981. *Introduction to Epstein-Barr Virus and Lymphoproliferative Diseases in Immunodeficient Individuals*. Cancer Research 41: 4209.

Qz202, G8750. 1983. *The Filterable Viruses*. Oncogenic Viruses, Vol. 1, Pergamon Press.

Rickinson, A.B., Moss, D.J., Wallace, L.E., Rowe, M., Misko, I.S., Epstein, M.A., and Pope, J.H. 1981, Nov. *Long-Term T-Cell-mediated Immunity to Epstein-Barr Virus*. Cancer Research 41: 4216–4221.

Rowley, Janet. 1982, 14 May. *Identification of the Constant Chromosome Regions Involved in Human Hematologic Malignant Disease*. Science (Wash. D.C.), 216: 749–750.

Saemundsen, A.K., Purtilo, D.T., Sakamoto, K., Sullivan, J.L., Synnerholm, A., Hanto, D., 1981, Nov. *Virus Infection in Immunodeficient Patients with Life-threatening Lymphoproliferative Diseases by Epstein-Barr Virus Complementary RNA/DNA and Viral DNA/DNA Hybridization.* Cancer Research 41: 4237–4242.

Shope, Richard E. 1932. *A Filtrable Virus Causing a Tumor-Like Condition in Rabbits and its Relationship to Virus Myxomatosum.* Journal of Experimental Medicine, 56: 803–822.

Shope, Thomas and Miller, George. 1973. *Epstein-Barr Virus: Heterophile Responses in Squirrel Monkeys Inoculated with Virus-Transformed Autologous Leukocytes,* Journal of Experimental Medicine, 137: 140–147.

Tosato, G., Macrath, I., Koski, I., Dooley, N., and Blaese, M. 1979, 22 Nov. *Activation of Suppressor T Cells During Epstein-Barr-Virus-Induced Infectious Mononucleosis.* The New England Journal of Medicine, 301: 1133–1137.

Trowell, H.C., and Burkitt, D.P. (editors). 1981. *Western Diseases. Their Emergence and Prevention.* London: Edward Arnold.

Trowell, H.C., Burkitt, D.P., and Heaton, K.W. (editors). 1985. *Dietary Fibre, Fibre—depleted Foods and Disease.* London: Academic Press.

West, Morris. 1981. *The Clowns of God.* London: Hodden and Stoughton.

Williams, E.H., Breslow. N.E., and Edlestein, R. 1982, Dec. *Results of Treatment of Burkitt's Lymphoma Patients in the West Nile District of Uganda at Kuluva Hospital.* East African Medical Journal, 785–792.

Wright, Dennis H. 1971. *Burkitt's Lymphoma: A Review of the Pathology, Immunology, and Possible Etiologic Factors.* Pathology Annual: 337–363.

****